Francisco Kaiut

JOURNEY TO
THE HEART OF PAIN

life story(ies) and the yoga that transforms (them)

a transversal narrative with
Edvaldo Pereira Lima

Journey to the Heart of Pain: life story (ies) and the yoga that transforms (them) - a transversal narrative with Edvaldo Pereira Lima.

Francisco Kaiut and Edvaldo Pereira Lima

Copyright © 2025 by Antonio Francisco Spercoski Kaiut and Edvaldo Pereira Lima.

ISBN 9786501327228

Published by Francisco Kaiut
Copy editing: Claire R. Chang
Design, layout, and cover: Israel Dias de Oliveira
Illustrations: Ednei Marx – Studio58

Translated by Edvaldo Pereira Lima from the Brazilian Portuguese original:
Viagem ao Coração da Dor: história de vida (s) e o yoga que a(s) transforma - uma narrativa transversal com Edvaldo Pereira Lima.

Contents

Truly Surreal

"As above, so below; as below, so above. As within, so without;
as without, so within. As big, so small; as small, so big. As
outside, so inside; as inside, so outside. The Whole lives in each
one; and each one belongs to the Whole."

The Principle of Correspondence,
attributed to Hermes Trismegistus

Three books in one. Three interwoven narratives. Three dynamic times—the past, the present, and a sign of the future. That's what you'll find here.

These narratives unfold across places near and far—Brazil, America, Europe, India, and Tibet—reflecting the borderless nature of timeless knowledge. They tell the story of one life and many entangled lives, a yoga method, and a Brazilian initiative of considerable influence. Together they culminate in a radically new knowledge that radiates from Brazil to the world.

All of this is occurring in a time of extraordinary transformation for our collective humanity, a time marked by dramatic challenges. It can seem that we are at a crossroads. On the one hand, there is pressure for society to advance towards a new milestone in civilization. However, our outdated models and limited perception of reality hold us back, leading to stagnation and even dangerous regression. These models and perceptions undermine our ability to see the extraordinary potential for individual and collective health that lies in the integration of body, mind, and heart.

A life of great potential awaits each of us. It calls us to take the courageous steps towards a majestic destination of empowerment, dignity, wonder, and perhaps, even happiness.

Simple as that. Complex like that.

At the center of everything is the human being. At the center of this journey is the protagonist,

Francisco Kaiut.

As Francisco navigates the swirling currents of his life, others cross his path. Many are trapped in a vortex of pain—pain that distorts reality, limits freedom, and can even extinguish the will to live. Yet this pain, in all its intensity, also acts as a compass and force that propels, pushes, pulls, and hurls people towards (re)discovering themselves, moving them towards unknown possibilities and untapped potential.

The route to access this journey of (re)discovery and hope?

The Kaiut Yoga method.

In the reflection of this mixed panorama of pain and suffering, and jubilation and hope, is you. Even if you don't recognize yourself in the scenery at first glance. Nothing happens by chance. Nothing.

As you are here, something of your being connects you with this field of knowledge, wisdom, and experience. You are already part of it, at least at the level of possibility. Just as the contemporary avant-garde sciences say, the wise traditions already said, and the visionary poets and artists have pointed out in the past and now, nothing is, in fact, isolated, fragmented, or hopelessly and forever separated from the delicately woven web of life that integrates everything and everyone.

So, this is an invitation.

You are invited to enter the mirror, abandon the passive comfort of the reflection, and embark on this journey. No need to knock on the door to this journey. The door is already open. You are welcome to join me as I shed light on the intriguing alchemical process of life, as exemplified by Francisco's journey. Together we will venture through pain and the folds of destiny that result in profound transformation and a very tangible and practical gift to the world—a path of liberation for countless others.

Who tells this story?

A symphony of voices. The main one is that of Francisco himself. Alongside him, are the voices of many real-life co-actors and co-authors of this great little epic. Then, guiding you through this journey is, I, Edvaldo, the writer, who weaves these narratives that combines thought and action, context and emotion.

We are all in the network of discoveries and challenges called life that propels us towards a possible evolution of consciousness that is dormant in our bodies. Movement is the key to awakening. And destiny may be more surprising than one imagines. Yet the outcome is not certain. Powerful obstacles are along the path— something Francisco knows all too well...

Our inner universe manifests the world around us. When I reflect on my story, I realize how much I lived in a rigid, reactive, traumatized universe. I want to be emotionally transparent with you, the reader, by sharing important times, places, and episodes of my journey.

This journey is not linear. It is complex, like life. Life can be traumatic. But it can also be fascinating. It depends on how you look at it. It depends on how much courage you muster to face what frightens you—those things in the past that persist in the mind, in the memory, in the emotions, but is also in the fibers and viscera of the present body of each one of us. Life can unleash potential you could only dream of, if, that is, you can face the monster that can make life miserable and limited: Pain.

1

Chiron's Gate

The invitation is for a journey. Like every journey, it is a call to adventure. Just like any adventure, it is a ticket for a deep dive with the promise of a treasure. And like any treasure hunt, there is a map with markings to orient and direct you but also symbols that require effort to decipher them. On this journey, finding the treasure requires questioning the beliefs that have shaped your mental model and perception of reality. You are challenged to open portals of perception that you might never have sought out were you not moved by the threat of suffering and the looming deterioration of your quality of life thanks to pain.

People are arriving. More than 70 are expected. The large majority are women. Many people are in their 40s and over, even in their 80s, some younger, 30 and under, and a five-month-old baby.

They come from different parts of Brazil, mostly from the South and Southeast, with one arriving from the United States. Joyful yet patient, they understand that this is just one chapter in a larger, systemic, ongoing process—one that is deeply connected to their innermost drive to live more fully. They recognize that this moment in their journey carries a clear purpose; part of their potential awakening to the greatness every human soul longs for and can ultimately achieve.

They know that the journey is inward. Their own. That the territory of adventure is their bodies. A very palpable territory. But they also know, that paradoxically, this material, physical world, that of the body, does not pulsate by itself. It is intertwined with the mind, with the nervous system, with the psyche, and with the emotions. But they need to (re)discover and (re)signify this in practice, in a very solid way, to free themselves from the societal constructs that have been imposed upon their minds, dictating not only who they are but what the world is and what things mean.

This is nothing stratospheric. There is nothing esoteric about this—there is no reason to be scared. The journey offers them a consistent path to navigate through this complexity, which is, in fact, everything that constitutes life. The path may seem counterintuitive if you look at it through the lens of distorted logic that prevails in society. But they are moved to unveil their hidden inner wisdom, the wisdom of nature that inhabits every human being. For this there is a need to dive underground into the unconscious, and not run away from what bothers them, disturbs them, controls them, and makes them suffer.

That's why they go down to the basement of the hotel, literally and metaphorically. They dive underground because it is here, in the Bromélia and Hortênsia rooms (names that refer to silently wise flora of nature), that their adventure takes place. Three days of intensive experience at the Kaiut Yoga Summit.

The word summit refers to the highest peak of a mountain. By association, it represents the high-level gathering of people interested in a specific topic. Here, the topic of interest is Kaiut Yoga, an extraordinarily transformative method of yoga created by Francisco Kaiut, developed in Brazil and expanded abroad.

Many of those who already know the method in the United States—and many of the people who are now entering the Summit—would say that the method is more than surprising, it is mind-blowing. It turns upside down the concept many people have of what yoga is. It radicalizes. In fact, Francisco criticizes part of classical, traditional yoga, pointing out the distortions of what he calls "off-the-shelf yoga", referring to commercialized, superficial, standardized, excluding approaches that currently have mass appeal. This powerful trend in North America was foolishly adopted in Brazil also; such cultural garbage masking the potential harm that "industrialized yoga fads" pose to our health.

The people who are here at the Summit already know that Kaiut Yoga has nothing to do with the performance of strange body positions that are designed, it seems, only for bodies with predispositions to acrobatic flexibility. These positions have the potential to cause serious structural damage even in bodies that can easily contort themselves into any shape.

That's why you see people arriving at the Summit wearing a t-shirt with an emblematic phrase of the method "Yoga for Everyone" (in Brazilian Portuguese, "Yoga Pra Tudo Mundo"). You don´t need to have the naturally gifted bodies of famous soccer players like Pelé or Marta in order to practice Kaiut Yoga. The method is for those of you who have never sat cross-legged on the floor, bending your body forward like an Indian fakir. It is for those of you who have never been interested in chanting a Hindu mantra. But also for those of you who practice Tibetan Buddhist meditation. It's for you, the professional athlete, who ruptured your tendon in the extreme exertion of high-performance sport. It's for you who are sedentary, who have never taken a brisk morning walk in the park around the corner. It's also for those of you who have walked the Camino de Santiago. The Kaiut Yoga Method is for everyone.

What brings these people from such different profiles and social and cultural conditions to be here?

Many are teachers of the method, and many others are just students.

But what unites them?

At the entrance to the Bromélia hall, a poster announces the Summit's intention, illuminating the participant's unifying interest: *Understanding Pain*.

This journey into pain at the Summit involves the delivery of knowledge, concepts, wisdom, and practice. For teachers of the method, the event supports them to guide their students on this provocative but fundamental journey. It is also for the teachers and students of the event to experience their own journey into pain.

The guide on this journey into pain?

Francisco himself.

He welcomes the participants with a friendly smile. He is wearing a black short-sleeved T-shirt with a visible "Ateliê São Paulo" pin. The term ateliê refers to a workspace for artistic or skilled creation, often with connotations of exclusivity and craftsmanship—fitting for Francisco's work. The pin also has his name and the logo of his brand, the letter K in gold surrounded by a circle, plus the phrase "Practitioner Since 3 Lives Ago".

Francisco has a solid, well-structured physical physique, with head, trunk, and limbs distributed in proportional harmony. He has none of the muscular exaggeration you would see in a competitive athlete. Francisco is 51 years old today. He has black hair with a few slightly gray strands. He stands at 5'9" (175 cm) tall and weighs around 147 lbs (67 kg).

At first glance, you don't find any trace of a show business-like charisma. Francisco does not exhibit an imposing ego presence; he doesn't display the exaggerated grandeur of a celebrity or show artificial extroverted behavior. One might expect these traits in someone who has attained success and fame.

In social moments, such as the reception, his presence is soft, more discreet, but friendly. Francisco speaks little and in short sentences, but you feel an intense presence when you notice him keenly focused on listening to whoever he is speaking with. It may break some of your hidden expectations. His expression is not what you might imagine of a celebrated Indian yoga guru, but the face of a kind-hearted fellow.

You may not initially see him as the soft, kind, and always smiling yoga teacher you might idealize in your dreams. Nor will you find the tough, iron-handed sergeant ready to punish you with a hundred push-ups if you miss a line of the national anthem. Equally absent is the vanity of a leader basking in the constant flattery from eager followers who idolize him.

But make no mistake. Francisco is indeed a master. As Carl Gustav Jung, the noble sage of human existence used to say, coincidences do not exist. Through the synchrony of life, Francisco is a master.

He is a master due to the precision of his life's purpose; the transparency with which he embraces his mission to serve others; the excellence with which he contributes to the practical improvement of the world and of people; and in the degree to which life allows all this to happen. Francisco is a master—without idolatry, but in all fairness and clarity.

You can only witness this master when he is engaged in his craft of excellence—teaching. In the social sphere, you may only see that Francisco is a nice guy, a good person, discreet, slightly friendly, but nothing out of the ordinary. You only notice the master's presence when you see him in action.

This Summit takes place in Gramado, the tourist heart of Serra Gaúcha, one of Brazil's most important tourism centers. The primary allure for tourists is the natural beauty of the region's mountains and forests, canyons, and ecological parks. Additionally, tourists come because of the cultural legacy of European immigration, especially Italian and German. The city of Gramado knows how to invest in tourism generating wealth for the city and surrounds. Tourism is the catalyzing center of economic prosperity here.

It is not by chance that Gramado is home to the only NASA (National Aeronautics and Space Administration) Theme Park in Brazil. It is also home to NBA (National Basketball Association) Park in Brazil; the NBA being the professional basketball league of the United States. The Park is the first entertainment-themed development of NBA in Brazil, with the gigantic leisure complex occupying almost one acre (4000 m^2).

The touristic aspects are not the primary reasons the Summit is taking place here in Gramado, however. The main reason is that Gramado has become an epicenter for the expansion of Kaiut Yoga in Brazil.

Francisco is from Curitiba, the capital of Paraná, 290 miles (468 kms) northwest of here. The metropolis is considered an exemplary urban model of sustainable development in Brazil. Francisco's work began in Curitiba, but its first spontaneous expansion took place in the state of Rio Grande do Sul, out of Gramado. The expansion was led by Camila Moscarelli, an early ally, a teacher of the method, and now, the local organizer of the Summit.

But why São Paulo on Francisco's pin?

Because he relocated to São Paulo, 694 miles (1118 kms) away from here. São Paulo is the country's central metropolis. It is a gigantic city with more than 12 million inhabitants as of 2023. It is the most influential Brazilian city on the global stage. In 2020 it ranked in the third level of the most globalized cities in the world, alongside metropolises such as Chicago, Frankfurt, Los Angeles, Toronto, Milan, and Amsterdam. São Paulo is now the base for Francisco's activities.

Those at the Summit know that to understand a teacher in the best sense of the word, it is necessary to open to the human complexity of such a remarkable person—in his greatness and in his fragility, in his glory and in his defeat. It is only from this more expansive perception that one can gain understanding of how such a person has become an inspiring and transformative leader, an exceptional teacher of teachers, and someone who transcends the noble function of teaching.

One of the instruments that can help us expand perception is the wisdom of Jung's humanistic psychology and its fusion with the richness of mythology. Jung's theory of archetypes gives us a way to understand the powerful psychic forces that circulate in the collective unconscious of humanity, while mythological narratives provide symbolic insight into the mysteries of life and the forces of the subtle world that collectively affect our lives.

How does this help us understand Francisco? What light does it shed on Francisco's choice to center the Summit on the subject of pain? Which is also a primary focus of his entire body of work.

Through the lenses of archetypes and mythology we can better understand what drives Francisco's life and his mission in the world. Mythological characters personify forces that embody possibilities, challenges, problems, and solutions, mirroring the dynamics of our lives. As archetypal models, they illuminate the motivations and needs underlying both individual and universal human experiences.

One of the most well-known mythological traditions comes from the classical period of Greek antiquity. Mythology from that time states that an infinity of diverse beings inhabited the superhuman Earth. Among them were gods and centaurs. Centaurs were mythological figures with a human head, torso, and arms, and the body of a horse. They were frequently depicted as violent, drunken beings, who caused confusion, chaos, and disturbance among the mythical pantheon.

But one of them had a different fate. Chiron was abandoned by his parents. This tragedy, let's say, a psychological one (if centaurs and gods had psyches), was actually a great blessing to him. The truth of things may not be what it appears at first glance.

Chiron was adopted by the god Apollo, who was the god of the arts, youth, and beauty, and versed in healing therapies and sciences.

In specific versions of the myth, Chiron was also adopted by the twin sister of Apollo, the goddess Artemis. Considered Apollo's spiritual wife, Artemis was a hunter but paradoxically was also the protector of animals, wild nature, women, and children. Raised under this privileged tutorship, Chiron had an education that we now call multidisciplinary, the integrated knowledge of various areas of expertise. As a result, he became an incredible mentor to many characters in Greek mythology and a renown healer.

One of his therapeutic feats involves Achilles. It turns out that this hero's mother, Thetis, wanted to make him immortal. To do this, she began burning Achilles' body and covering it with mug wort. His father, Peleus, didn't like this at all. He took Achilles from his mother's hands before she could complete the work and gave him to Chiron to educate him.

When he received young Achilles, Chiron realized that the child's heel was burned, an area where his mother had not had time to apply the therapeutic balm of mug wort. Saddened by the boy's suffering, Chiron placed a giant bone at the site of the wound, giving rise to this expression that would cross eras, peoples, and nations—"Achilles' heel"—which most people use without knowing its meaning.

But where does Chiron's compassion for others come from? What is the origin of his propensity towards educating, healing, and helping others?

One day, Chiron was in battle against the centaurs, alongside his friend and disciple Heracles, a demigod of extraordinary physical strength. Chiron, a profound connoisseur of herbs, prepared a poisoned arrow for his friend. At the height of chaotic fighting, Heracles, perhaps confusing Chiron with the other centaurs, unintentionally hit him with the poisoned arrow, in his thigh just above the knee. The poison is potent, but since Chiron is immortal, it cannot kill him. But it generates a brutal pain, which he could not erase, even with his vast therapeutic knowledge. The only relief he finds is to dedicate himself to healing others, moved by the high degree of empathy and compassion he develops.

This myth represents, in Jung's language, the archetype of the "Wounded Healer". It is an archetype available to the collective. A pattern of behavior that can manifest in an individual's life, which the individual can embrace and act on depending on the degree of self-awareness that he can achieve.

Where is Francisco in all this?

He was also wounded by a poisoned arrow in childhood. A modern arrow—in his case is a gunshot—that unleashed a pain that would change his life forever.

He tells this story himself later on. What he is exercising today at the opening of the Summit in Gramado is the compassionate result from this traumatic episode of his past. This outcome of compassion is woven together with his experience and deep knowledge of the art and science he developed to launch people toward their own stories of Chiron. In the first hours of the Summit, you hear him in his serene but firm style, without great emphatic fanfare of tone, speak to this journey towards Chiron.

I wish you a lot of pain throughout the whole event. No therapeutic process does not go through the heart of pain. That's why I don't want anyone to be painless. We don't relieve anyone's pain. What we do is activate Nature to reactivate the rescue gear, but for this, you must keep the ego from getting in the way of the process. And then you can live without pain.

It's easy to repeat Francisco's words. But in practice it is not so easy. The first step is to go toward and get in touch with the pain. The journey is exclusively yours. No one can do it for you. People here know that. But they also know that, paradoxically, facing their demons of pain and suffering is, in fact, not a solitary, lonely journey. Because no one is alone, really, on this ultimate venture. No one embarks on their adventure of transformation disconnected from the systemic fields that constitute the episodes of a life in motion. We are all intertwined. Our destinies intersect the paths of others, forming the same journey on different planes, collective and individual, crossing times and spaces.

People here know that. They participate in the living history of Francisco and the method, encountering along the way other allies who are also contributing to its co-creation.

Those allies include Ravi, Francisco's son. At 26 years of age, he is calm, with a more extroverted temperament than his father. Tattoos are scattered all over his body, some visible on his arms under a short-sleeved shirt. He is also a host of the Summit, teacher of the method, and the executive of a new phase of expansion of Kaiut Yoga in Brazil and around the world. Antonio is Francisco's father. At 83 years of age, he is equally engaged in the process. A teacher-curator who will conduct a key lecture on longevity, unpacking a topic associated with the central theme of pain. Both have their respective stories of Chiron, those of physical pain and pain of the soul, which ultimately are dynamic processes of the same underwater bed of reality integrated into the unconscious, needing to come to the surface.

Alissa, Francisco's wife, has a soft presence, eyes bright with excitement for the method and Kaiut Yoga. She plays a vital role behind the scenes, helping to anchor the mission in São Paulo. She is a force of action, hidden in her petite frame. Bruna, Ravi's wife, is a young teacher and ally of her husband and father-in-law. She exudes a freshness of youthful maturity that impresses this writer. Bento, Francisco's first grandson, sometimes rests serenely in his grandfather's arms, as he circulates around the room.

You will get to know many more allies of this story as this narrative unfolds. Many are students who are not teachers of the method, but are immersed in the Summit, aware of how just important the event is for them to learn how to become masters in facing their own challenges with Chiron. They seem to have made an implicit pact with Francisco, responding to his provocation in the Summit materials distributed to the participants:

What if, in life, movement was as necessary as food?

This provocation is woven into Francisco's speeches that are delivered throughout the event in conceptual talks, interactive question-and-answer sessions, and during practice. The starting point is the question of mobility. Nature sculpted the human body to move freely. However, modern civilization—rooted in unnatural self-indulgence, mercantilist priorities, and reductionistic, mechanistic worldviews—stifles these capacities. These forces immobilize, atrophy, harm and sicken the body. Worse, modern society distorts and hides the harm it causes, manipulating our minds, camouflaging the truth, and masking the problem of pain.

Guys, look at that. Some of you are surprised at the level of discomfort that I generate in you or reveal to exist within you. It seems like a scary thing...

But check it out, everyone has a brain that has learned to desire things. Wishing is the nature of being alive. What do you want? When you open your eyes in the morning, you want to get out of bed. So, if you desire to get up, your system can't reveal your problems. The brain is moved by desires. It is a wish box, like Aladdin's lamp.

If you wish to stand, walk, or take your grandchild or child in your arms, and have the life you dream of having, your brain will use all possible compensatory routes so that you don't realize that your neck is crooked, and that your body's labyrinth system—the complex system in the inner ear that is responsible for hearing and balance—is toasted. You already have a labyrinth condition; it just hasn't become symptomatic yet. You already have a rotten hip; you just don't have pain yet. Because there are still possible compensatory routes.

At some point though, the compensatory routes will dry up. When we have used them all, pain will be inevitable. Then, the cycle of frustration will begin.

When the student is led to feel significant limitations, this perception of limitations speaks to his most profound nature.

Take for example what happened here, with Lara's shoulder problem. I communicated to her that,

"This crap here has been hidden for decades. Whenever you do downward dog in conventional yoga—which is itself like dog training—you hurt that shoulder more."

When you bring people face to face with their pain, they realize that it does not belong to them. And they are delighted with the possibility of getting rid of it.

When we avoid noticing, we get sick.

My student from São Paulo, Roberta, thought she had a sciatic nerve problem and a back problem that was born from the sedentary lifestyle at the time of the COVID-19 pandemic. But that's not it.

There is a difference in the length of her legs. There is a story of a body sitting, working, disconnected so that the mind can operate on the computer. So, I didn't want to take away her pain.

What is it to relieve her back pain?

Back pain is irrelevant. Back pain can go away, even with an injection. It's not that it solves the pain, but the pain disappears. Now, if I can travel back in time to when this pain didn't exist, then I've made a therapeutic process exist there.

This is a process of rescue. The delivery of this rescue requires communication and education. Through communication and education, I can lead a student to a more intelligent understanding— not intellectualization—of their situation, of their pain and wish to escape it, such that they eventually arrive in a place thinking, "Man, I don't want to live with this awful situation anymore!"

Of course, the experience of rescue and removing what doesn't belong in your system is almost like an exorcism, like in that old movie, The Exorcist...

Everyone laughs with Francisco.

You cry. Your head turns inside out. It takes work.

But is it better to do that than to let these issues run wild inside you? What do you choose? What makes someone feel old, if not the lack of security to stand up?

The feeling of helplessness, of incapacity, is brutal. You can keep pretending and doing everything you wanted up until yesterday. But when those feelings of lack of security, or hopelessness comes, you despair. And such emotional shock can be enormous.

Everyone wants to find out what doesn't work. They just don't know that this possibility exists.

The student wants to find out the real reason for their pain and issues. Lara was led to believe that being upside down and doing downward dog was the sole cause of her pain, but then she discovered that it was not this. She discovered that it was something else. She stayed there, and she jumped up, and she jumped down, and she jumped up, and she jumped down. This did tear up her shoulder!

However, she also came to understand the block and limitation in her system existed before any downward dog,

"My god, how long has this thing been here?"

At that point, there was no doubt. There is no doubt, people. People just need to be introduced to my logic.

But to find the intrinsic coherence in Francisco's logic often requires turning your head inside out, in more than one direction. For Summit participants, through practicing together and sharing their experiences, they help each other comprehend Francisco's logic. It can also be useful to look at where Francisco's logic diverges from the big business world of conventional yoga and where it conflicts with the commodified health industry that also currently shapes the yoga world. Slowly, but surely, the logical foundations of Francisco's approach become clear.

Francisco´s and Kaiut Yoga's journey is not paved by a bed of roses. Thorns and dangers line the road. This Summit is a good portal. But it's just the beginning.

Come along. Turning your mind and body inside out may also be for you.

2

Our Daily Pain

W*e need to be very intimate with these areas that are suffering and that scare us. There is no path to rescuing the body and mind that does not pass through the middle of what scares us the most. There is no way out of chronic, joint, or highly complex pain that does not involve the experience of pain.*

Let's make peace with what scares us, with areas of sensitivity, and with strong sensations. There is no way out of anxiety that does not pass through acceptance of anxiety. The process of aging well calls for proactivity. Aging needs to be processed; it needs to be assimilated. There are people who choose to grow up without embracing the idea of maturing. This only generates more pain and suffering.

Doing yoga is about acceptance—maturity and acceptance.

Doing yoga is a game for grown-ups.

Francisco moves through the Summit with authenticity and a rightful ownership of his role as mentor for this group of people who have become an extension of his work, many of them also touched by the trials and tribulations of their own Chiron journeys. Each person here experiences, in their own way, the effects of the procedures and techniques of Kaiut Yoga under the watchful eye and guidance of the method's creator. They also cultivate their own roles as educators and guides to healing. They dialogue with each other and Francisco, sharing success stories and intriguing and challenging cases from their students, or themselves.

Francisco is judicious in sharing the solid theoretical basis of his work. However, he best demonstrates the coherent and expressive harmony between theory and practice when he leads the dynamic activities of the event.

In the Hortênsia room, participants, as they sit on their mats, have at their disposal a series of accessories designed for the best possible engagement with practice. Red bolsters—cylindrical cushions to accommodate head and body in various positions— are strategically positioned on each mat. Wooden wedges for the feet are there to support positions that, in the method, defy the conventional logic of balancing bodies. Black straps wait for their time to help maintain stability and posture.

None of this is unique to the method. They are classic yoga accessories. However, when you investigate the principles, purpose, and guiding intent that Francisco gave to his creation, Kaiut Yoga has little similarity with other approaches to this ancient practice of yoga.

Too often, we sit on the mat and jump into the first action without realizing the reality of the moment, without allowing ourselves to perceive patterns of anxiety, insecurity, and discomfort. The practice then risks becoming a distraction and not a moment of yoga itself, in its deepest sense.

Fear, pain, doubt, all these must be brought to the mat and processed throughout the practice.

From here, the body begins to bother you. The hips start to bother you. The back starts to bother you. And that's okay.

Noticing this, also perceive not you breathing, but this phenomenon of Nature breathing for you, providing everything. Noticing this, very slowly, bend forward. More sensations will arise, be in contact with them. Contact! Get out of doing it and come to feel it. Feel the hip. Feel any tension or rigidity. Feel any disconnection. Identify all these patterns.

This disconnection to our hips often negatively impacts pelvic and spine health. Just feel it. Reorient your dynamics. There is no achievement, no effort. There is perceiving, and there is allowing the body to show itself as it really is.

Within the pelvis, the head of the femur turns outwards, causing the entire pelvic structure to rotate on top of the femur heads, leading to an initial forward curvature of the spine. Of course this results in a gradual increase of sensation. But you can manage the sensation.

If it starts to hurt too much, you can move your torso back a little. You can have a certain sense of control, that is very important. The sense of control gives you the ability to keep your own nervous system feeling safer. That way, you will trust the position, the work, and the approach more.

With all this happening, go back to perceiving breathing. Perceive Nature itself as providing flow, providing... life! So, get out of that place of perfect, ideal, controlled breathing.

Don't judge. I breathe well, I breathe badly, I don't know how to breathe. Forget all that. Get out of that place and go to the experience. You don't need to have any sense of control of breathing. The phenomenon of breathing happens in many ways. It can be a consequence of our emotions and anxieties. It can be an exercise in control that stiffens the mind. Or it may just be a phenomenon of Nature itself... Nature within us! Regulating the nervous system, supporting emotional balance, and providing metabolic health. Release this breath that simply occurs. Feel the rhythm of this breath spreading throughout the entire system.

Just feel it. Just allow it. Just feel it.

Do yoga from a very different perspective. Get out of the action, get out of control, get out of the effort. Enter into the experience of this feeling that generates the meditative state. Eyes closed... a breath that breathes itself.

We talk a lot about the mind-body connection. In fact, there is neither mind nor body. It's all one thing. What we want, through practice, is a smarter body, a body that thinks on its own, and a brain that doesn't think when it's not needed or when it isn't productive.

Let it all appear. Take yourself to a new place. Take yourself to new, different, and unfamiliar spaces.

For some, there is already a lot of pain. Guys, what is this pain?

That pain already lives inside you. And the function of practice is to take it from there. It is recreating an experience and a detoxification process. All rigidity has a toxic consequence. Every position has a detoxifying effect.

The room is in absolute silence, except for a soothing murmur of running water synchronously beginning to flow in a small garden feature just outside one of the windows. Then there is Francisco's voice that intermittently breaks the silence.

The ambient climate is serene. The subtle atmospheric field that envelops space makes it seem that time itself has stretched, moving at a peaceful rhythm. It's slow living. A slow life. A balsamic breath. The air that enters through your nostrils sharpens your sense that something very subtle, but nourishing is actually feeding you... that external life is pulsating in you...

Francisco's movements do not generate any noise. He doesn't stand in a fixed point. He walks slowly, discreetly throughout the space of the Hortênsia room, observing every minute detail. It is as if his body were a radar antenna picking up environmental signals.

Here, he is like a sun that triggers the galactic spin of planets, seeking to awaken each person to the awareness of their own individual spins and that of the simultaneous collective cosmic dance that orchestrates everything—the parts and the whole.

He is a conductor who manages the harmony of the ensemble while maintaining a sharp perception of the momentum of each instrument. He knows that there is only one music. Yet he remains aware of the thousands of distinct sounds that can potentially arise from the musicians and his own self. He, along with them, is enveloped by an immanent, all-encompassing symphony—a presence that seems omniscient, guiding and connecting everything in its vast, harmonious embrace.

With your eyes closed, come back slowly.
Closed... Ana Paula!
Guys, that's it. We try to take a peek. We try to control the environment. Our anxiety patterns want to take control of our life

experiences. Anxiety wants to make itself more anxious at every moment. It would help if you put a short leash on it. It would help if you took control.

You have to peek inside. Pause slowly, deeply. Let the entire rhythm disassemble. Put your body, mind, heart, and everything on pause. Learn about limits and being constructive in dealing with weaknesses.

When it comes to our pain, we feel, look, welcome, and investigate its essence. Where does it come from? How intense is it?

Only then can we process it. Only then can we enter a therapeutic process and dissolve it.

You cannot get there through being aggressive. It requires working with depth. Working in this place where I like to take you, and you like to be taken, requires kindness.

Time passes extended and slow. Francisco's voice resonates calmly, the tone conveying an implicit message that you are safe here. He is attentive to the collective group but also to each one, to you.

Come back, legs crossed. Very good!
That's it, Flávia.
Turn that heel inward, Claudia!
It's ok, it's ok there, Georgina!
A peak of pressure, Norberto!

The notion of time is precise. Room management is one of Francisco's didactic masteries. In this practice, he is delivering one of his more spontaneously developed classes—it unfolds movement by movement, position by position, in a sequence that is coherent with the logic of the method.

There are a total of 100 foundational classes in the method. Each teacher in the training course receives the written scripts of these classes to deliver themselves. But they are not a straitjacket. Kaiut Yoga is not performance. It is presence.

Each student is accompanied by Francisco's sharp gaze strolling through the room. His simultaneous radar sweep of individuals and the collective is very rare to see in any teaching situation in any field of knowledge.

How long should the student be left in a position, even when their discreet moans of pain run through the room? Why is the girl in the blue sweatshirt instructed to cross her legs from a sitting position directly on the mat, while the mature gentleman in a white shirt and gray hair is instructed to sit in the same positions but on the red bolster?

Experiment with everything. Ahah ... ahah... Very good, people. Immerse yourself in the sensation. Stay with it.

Pause. Silence. Restrained moans. Francisco approaches a participant. He crouches down next to her. He says something and touches her upper back lightly. He comments to the group:

She doesn't like this leg position. It's like taking cod liver oil...

A collective laugh echoes through the room. When the participants stand up, feet on the wedges, they bend their bodies forward and stay there for what seems like endless minutes, which calls for more humor:

It is the detachment of the fascia. Let it all dissolve. Don't let the nervous system get stressed out, for Shiva's sake! This is not physical activity.

A rebellious moan and a barely camouflaged whisper emerge here and there, three or four participants letting the experience of their pain express itself. More humor:

Come on, guys, it's ending! It's ending. What's ending? This incarnation!

And then the final catharsis:

Now, walk—without running away from the sensation. Let the body reset the experience. Let the brain reorganize around what has happened.
Roberta, walk a little.
Celso, walk a little.

The practices and conceptual talks throughout the event are activities that are very dear to the participants, especially to teachers of the method. Then there are case presentations that reinforce confidence or allow teachers to correct their inevitable mistakes. They cherish the opportunity to receive supervision from the collective and the person who created all this.

They too are seeking mastery, hopeful that it comes with practice, from the analysis of cases, and from the first-hand knowledge directly from the source, which they can then incorporate in their teaching roles.

The more spine and hip surgeries that men undergo, the more prostate cancer we have. Everything that moves a man's pelvis will move the prostate. The prostate is driven by pelvic floor health.

Am I against surgery?

No, I'm not. If you need surgical intervention, have it. However, you stop integrating the emotional side of things, which will just create issues is in the long-term. Modern medicine starts from a totally incorrect initial perspective, the perspective of segmentation, and not of rescue. We stop being an animal with a paw and become a super sophisticated modern being that never put our foot on the ground without shoes.

Here we have Michael, who spends a lot of time on his bike. To pedal he has a pedalboard where he locks in his shoe allowing him to generate power. Essentially though, it means he doesn't have a functional foot when on his bike. The pedalboard locks all circuits. He pedals well. But when he's finished, he gets off the bike. How?

Like every cyclist...

Francisco makes funny, crookėd body movements and walks a little gangly. Everyone laughs, even Michael, a tall, athletic man looking just over 50 years old, with a body that looks like it's been built through sport.

And what does this do to him in the medium term?

That little foot, with its abundance of nerve endings—more than even the hands—begins to fade from the brain's map through lack of use. This fading erases the brain's primary tool for balance and stability. The brain requires a highly functional foot to support its balancing mechanisms effectively.

The labyrinthine system, central to our ability to balance and orient ourselves in space, is designed to work in synergy with the feet—tools of extraordinary technological sophistication, refined by Nature. When these tools are underused or impaired, they become weakened, leaving the brain without its essential partner for balance. In response, the brain attempts to compensate, but these compensations often lead to misalignments and, ultimately, pain.

Do you understand the compensatory routes?

So, the subject of yoga practice is rescue. As a species, we were made to walk miles and miles a day. We weren't made for "training."

The nature of our species is adaptability. Yet, in modern society, adaptability is precisely what we've lost. We now have advanced mattresses, high-tech pillows—even ones designed by NASA—yet many of us still sleep poorly. Why?

Because the environment of modern life adapts itself entirely to us, while we fail to adapt to anything. This lack of adaptability undermines one of the core engines of our species' health and vitality. Adaptability is what drives us, what nourishes us, and it exists in every joint, every tissue, and every structure of our bodies.

So, what is practice?

Practice is the place to rescue adaptability.

Oh, that's fine, but what about knee pain?

The pain isn't just about the knee. It's the knee desperately screaming because you no longer have a healthy, functional foot to support it, or well-functioning hips to stabilize it.

Do you understand?

The body's pain is often its way of signaling that its interconnected systems have lost their natural adaptability; has no more compensatory routes. Practice is the key to restoring that.

Many people in the room understand. It sinks in for those who have not yet realized the intertwined logic of facts and situations that sustain the foundations of the method from a dynamic, systemic, holistic, holographic perspective. Everything is integrated, life is relational and processual, and everything is distributed in a dynamically wise way in Nature. We are the ones who lose focus, falling into the reductionism of the current mental models that tend to fragment our perception of reality, reducing it to an overly simplistic angle that distorts the whole nature of what existence is, what life is, and what our bodies are. Just as they corrupt our conception of what old age and aging are.

Pain, the central theme of this Summit, is associated, at Kaiut Yoga, with the issue of health, which has everything to do with longevity. This is the theme addressed by Antonio Kaiut, Francisco's father. He is a very appropriate speaker for this speech, both due to his work as a health professional, his blood connection with Francisco and his son's work, and his personal condition.

At 83 years old, the widower of Lucy, Francisco's mother, Antonio is married to Ana, almost 50 years younger, with whom he has a son, Mahari, now 12 years old. A renowned masseuse, chiropractor, and former military policeman, Antonio draws smiles of approval from the audience in the middle of his speech.

The issue in our society is the view that being elderly inevitably involves suffering, pain, and an inability to care for oneself. But I wonder if it has to be that way. Let's get it out of our heads that the older person is finished, has no chance in life, and has to sit in a corner and take medicine.

Last week, the press reported that actor Al Pacino became a father for the fourth time at 83. But we have a champion in this matter. It's not me...

Laughter erupts from the group.

It is an Indian man who became a father for the second time at 96, having been for the first time at 94. They asked this gentleman what the secret was. He replied that he kept himself healthy and that he enjoyed sex with his wife.

I agree with him. I think it's essential for husband and wife to have sex regularly. For my part, I care about my wife. I give her what she needs. She is a pleased woman!

Antonio's recipe for longevity is composed of a triangle with healthy living at one vertex (which includes correct nutrition and sex) and the cultivation of good humor and memory at another. The third vertex is spirituality, faith in something greater than ourselves.

In this context, Kaiut Yoga is a yoga school focused on health promotion. Ravi later emphasizes this in his talk. He also offers insight into how the method is positioned in the contemporary global yoga scene.

Yoga has become an ever-expanding worldwide phenomenon and a major industry, generating billions of dollars annually in the United States alone. Unsurprisingly then, this has been one place for Kaiut Yoga's international expansion, with its roots firmly planted in North America for years. This event in Gramado, however, marks a significant moment for the Kaiut community. For the Kaiuts, it represents a historical milestone in the method's development—leveraging its impact in Brazil and solidifying the first phase of its national expansion.

The event celebrates the foundation of a strong, dedicated community of teachers and practitioners who share a collective vision. These individuals are not just participants but co-creators of a long-term journey of continuous renewal and evolution. Ravi eloquently highlights this shared dream and the promising future it holds, inspiring all those in attendance.

The strongest trend in the market today is the presentation of yoga as a health method. Research shows this. It's a very different idea from what the concept of yoga was in the 1970s, especially in the United States. The Americanization of yoga greatly influenced Brazil and other countries, selling yoga as a physical activity. "I'm going to do yoga to have more toned abs, less fat on my body, and to be stronger."

But those who seek yoga today want health. The veteran teachers in America are the ones who mostly ignored this change in the public. However, a small group of young teachers in the United States understood the change. Therefore, the idea of selling yoga as a therapeutic health process is already widespread. That's where Kaiut Yoga comes in. But in what context? There is a big competition between everyone in this market nowadays.

Yoga, as an industry, is *big* business.

There are 300 million people who practice yoga worldwide, of which 72% are women, according to a 2023 survey by Gitnux in New York, a company specializing in monitoring consumer trends in various sectors. India is the country with the highest number of practitioners, 191 million, while Brazil, according to Ravi's survey, has one million practitioners. Compare that to the United States which has about 55 million practitioners, with about 14 million of those practitioners over 50 years of age. Around 39,000 establishments—schools and studios—offer yoga and Pilates classes in the United States, with more than 55,000 yoga teachers registered in the country.

When you look at the economic data, the numbers are equally impressive. The yoga industry—comprising manufacturers of accessories, equipment, and other materials for the practice—is an 84-billion-dollar global market. It is expected to grow by 9.6% per year until 2027, with the United States leading the expansion and followed by countries in the Asia-Pacific. The global market for yoga clothing and attire had a market value of 6.38 billion dollars in 2020, while the entirety of the yoga sector–schools and studios plus the industry–estimated at 106 billion dollars.

No Wall Street capitalist would fault such business. It's an eye-opener for big investors.

The commodification of the practice, led by the North American industry, distorts the original purpose of yoga, as Francisco has spoken to. Ravi however shares a timeline for to understand the changes that have occurred in trends and proposals over the years, and what Kaiut Yoga is navigating.

The method aims to redefine the practice of yoga—not as a form of physical exercise, but as a health practice, a way to optimize the body and mind through natural tools that have been largely forgotten or neglected in modern life. This vision presents a unique challenge because it still involves engaging the body, which society predominantly associates with fitness and exercise.

We face the task of providing substantial education to distinguish our approach to yoga from two dominant paradigms that shape public perception: the religious framework, brought from India to the West, and the American "fitness yoga" trend. Both have heavily influenced how yoga is understood today.

However, the original concept of yoga was far broader. Archaeological evidence from over three thousand years ago, uncovered in India, reveals that yoga was designed to engage the whole body, integrating physical, mental, and spiritual dimensions. Our method seeks to reconnect with this holistic vision, offering a modern application of yoga as a practice rooted in health and well-being rather than religion or fitness culture.

Ravi emphasizes that health is at yoga's origin. The dominant classical lines of practice, such as Hatha, Vinyasa, Iyengar, and Ashtanga, have this commitment at their root.

Where did the distortion start then?

In Indian antiquity, Patañjali is regarded as the first scholar to systematize and codify the knowledge of yoga into written literature. Before this, yoga teachings were likely passed down orally from generation to generation. Patañjali compiled this knowledge in the form of the Yoga Sutras, associating it with sacred Hindu texts such as the Puranas, Vedas, and Upanishads.

Many centuries later, yoga reached the West for the first time when the monk Swami Vivekananda delivered a landmark presentation on yoga at the First Parliament of Religions in Chicago in September 1893. This event established a lasting association between yoga, Hinduism, and religion in the Western imagination. Vivekananda spent years traveling across North America and Europe, sharing teachings on yoga within the framework of Hindu philosophy.

Vivekananda was a disciple of Paramahamsa Ramakrishna, a pivotal religious leader of the late nineteenth century, known for his profound influence on Indian cultural renewal. This movement of spiritual revival continued into the twentieth century, gaining greater momentum after India's independence in 1947. With independence, yoga began to evolve beyond its medieval ascetic and monastic traditions. It entered a phase of modernization, with teachers adapting and reimagining yoga to fit contemporary contexts, including dialogues with Western science to highlight its health benefits.

One of the early pioneers in this transformation was Sri Yogendra, a disciple of Vivekananda, who established a yoga teaching center in 1918. His goal was to present yoga from a scientific perspective. In 1929, Swami Kuvalayananda introduced a postgraduate course in yoga that integrated insights from physiology and Western medicine, attracting students from around the world. By 1936, Swami Sivananda Saraswati, a trained physician, opened a study center that blended medical research with the subtle spiritual insights found in texts like the Bhagavad Gita to explain yoga's principles.

In parallel, Sri Tirumalai Krishnamacharya, an Ayurvedic doctor, revitalized yoga by drawing on the teachings of his master, Ramamohana Brahmacharya, who lived as a hermit in a Himalayan cave. Krishnamacharya brought this ancient wisdom into a modern India that was growing in cultural self-confidence during its struggle for independence from British rule. His innovative approach shaped a generation of influential disciples who adapted classical yoga to contemporary needs, ensuring its global consolidation.

These disciples included Bellur Krishnamachar Sundararaja Iyengar (B.K.S. Iyengar), who focused on perfecting asanas (yoga postures) and developed practice tools and techniques specifically suited to Western practitioners, creating a lineage that bears his name. K. Pattabhi Jois developed Ashtanga Vinyasa Yoga, a dynamic and physically demanding style, while T.K.V. Desikachar introduced Viniyoga.

In another vein, the monk Paramahansa Yogananda, heir to another ancient lineage called Hatha Yoga, made an extraordinary contribution to the popularization of yoga in the West. Renaming it Kriya Yoga, he blended the religious traditions of Hinduism with what he termed the "yoga of Jesus." Settling in California, Yogananda gained the admiration of prominent figures in science, business, and entertainment, including George Eastman (founder of Kodak), actress Greta Garbo, and conductor Leopold Stokowski.

In the 1960s, parallel to the counterculture movement, yoga entered a new phase of expansion in North America. Over the next decade, yoga's proponents began to strip away the mystical and religious connotations that once accompanied it. Gradually, yoga penetrated the mainstream, becoming part of the cultural fabric of American society. However, this transition came at a cost. In Francisco's view, yoga fell into the trap of high-consumption culture, which commodifies everything for superficial comfort. This transformation gave rise to "fitness yoga," detaching the practice from its original connection to health and well-being. Yoga was reduced to a means of achieving a fit body, often overlooking the fact that improper practice could harm the body, causing injuries and rendering it less functional.

Ravi's speech at the Summit sheds light on the context in which Kaiut Yoga is situated and the challenges it faces in Brazil and around the world. It also highlights the obstacles Francisco had to overcome to establish Kaiut Yoga as a groundbreaking method. Through his efforts, the method has gained remarkable traction globally, redefining yoga's purpose and its approach to health.

Today, the impact of Kaiut Yoga is undeniable. As of the beginning of 2025, there are sixteen licensed Kaiut Yoga schools across Brazil, including Francisco's headquarters in São Paulo. In the United States, there are another nine licensed schools, one in Portugal and one in Italy. The method has associated 131 teachers in Brazil, 128 in the United States, more than 3000 certified teachers around the world, including Canada, Germany, South Africa, the Netherlands, Portugal, Italy, Australia and more than 50,000 practitioners worldwide—these numbers growing each year. The method reflects 35 years of continuous practice and development.

In addition to its physical presence, Kaiut Yoga has expanded into the digital sphere with online teacher training courses, live classes in English, and digital courses for practitioners. The Kaiut Health app has extended the method's reach, now available on over a thousand devices. Post-pandemic, the number of students doubled in both Curitiba and São Paulo, signaling the method's increasing relevance and effectiveness. These results include countless cases of transformative experiences, with teachers and students alike learning to navigate and transcend their pain— Francisco and Ravi included. Many of these stories will be shared throughout this narrative.

The challenges faced by Francisco and the method are far from simple. They include breaking the longstanding association of yoga with religion and mysticism, countering its framing as a mere fitness activity, and introducing an avant-garde approach that forces people to think outside the box and confront deeply ingrained paradigms. As Francisco himself explains, there are even more hurdles to address.

Let's say, the person has improved significantly, and pain has decreased—so let's stop?

No. I prefer to give more space for Nature itself to solve the problem. I'm not a fan of using anything that sedates a person. We already live in a society that is, in many ways, sedated. People engage in excessive physical activity, thinking it will solve their problems, but it often only increases their anxiety.

I see it clearly in the United States. By the time people reach 70, many who have overexerted themselves physically are dealing with bodies that are worn down. They're anxious, relying on medication to sleep and suffering from more chronic pain than those who have been sedentary. Why? Because at 40, no one asked them, "Jack, why are you running so much? Why are you eating so much? Is it out of concern for your overall health, or is it fear of becoming obese? Have you considered that this approach might lead to trouble down the road?"

The anxiety we're trying to address doesn't go away with physical exhaustion—it's solved through methods like meditation, not overexertion. Physical exhaustion might knock you out at night when you're 40, and maybe even at 50 or 60. But by the time you're 70, your body can't keep up with that cycle anymore. The habit of relying on exhaustion to sleep leaves your mind trapped, anxious, and unable to remember what a natural, restorative night's sleep even feels like.

That's not what we want. Our goal is to help students awaken their own innate systems, to let Nature step in and regenerate. It's not about forcing something to happen; it's about creating the conditions for Nature's own mechanisms to come back online. That's the core idea—nothing else.

Is it difficult? Of course. It's not easy. A practice like today's dismantles your entire way of being. Why? Because true relaxation is terrifying for many people. Today, I guided you into a practice where everyone lay still on the mat. And what happened? In that stillness, the world as you know it seemed to vanish. At the peak of your anxiety, you faced something uncomfortable: the absence of compulsive thinking. That moment is unsettling. It's scary. But it's also the beginning of something transformative.

This question we need to ask here is: what is natural health?

This Summit, now drawing to a close, has been driven by the collective search for answers—a quest sparked by the universal experience of pain.

As we turn the page, let us embark together on a journey into the past, exploring this story and its history, adventuring into unfamiliar and inhospitable terrain. It is the story of a man whose encounter with pain became the catalyst for finding a purpose that gives his life meaning. Like Chiron, the wounded healer, he forges a new path—one that holds the potential to guide many others.

Yet, as with any act of renewal, this journey must confront the entrenched, crystallized shadows that obscure life. These shadows manifest not only in the structures of society but also in the recesses of our minds and hearts, challenging the clarity and courage required to move forward.

3

A Shot at the Dawn of Life

*I*was playing with my cousin Carlos. I was six. He was seven. We were in the backyard of his house in Curitiba. We were joking around... having fun playing good guy and bad guy... shooting at each other with toy guns... like we saw in the Western movies on television... a very 1970s thing.

My father stopped by to pick me up. That day he had left work and gone to the farm of my uncle Fausto, his brother, outside the city. This uncle of mine needed help with land grabbers and land ownership issues. It was a different time then in Brazil, a time of the military dictatorship, yet a lot of rural violence. My father was a captain in the Military Police.

The whole family was military. Several, if not all of my uncles, were military. My father was already in a prominent position in his career. He was well respected in the field. He had gone to the

United States to take training courses. He was assigned to work at the National Information Service, the dictatorship's espionage agency. He was also a professor of mathematics and physics at the Military College of Curitiba, a very charismatic guy among the students, and a strict and dedicated professional.

It was a family that had faced financial hardships and extreme domestic violence in the past. Carlos's father, my uncle Renê, was married to aunt Cássia, who is my father's sister. Renê was an aggressive man and also served as an officer in the Military Police.

I think that because of the origin of a family like this, my father was very limited in his ability to express emotions. He was restrained. He was never physically or verbally violent with me, his only son, nor with my mother, Lucy. He was not abusive in any way. He was, provocative. That's what he was. His approach reflects a language rarely seen today, one where challenge is used as a tool to educate. But where he came from, it was the only way. He became a brilliant father of a child in his own way. But in his family of origin, aggression was intense.

The home of my uncle Fausto, who had also been in the military, was filled with conflict. He had a problem with alcoholism. He beat dogs, sometimes his wife, and his son. Think of a woman being beaten with a dog chain, blood splashing everywhere. Another uncle of mine burned my cousin's hands on a hot plate on a wood stove as punishment for something.

I felt very privileged because, in my nuclear family, there was no such thing, but a certain degree of violence permeated around me. It was an insane thing. If there was any violence from my father at home, it was to cover up that of his brothers. It shocked me a lot when he showed this aspect of him.

I think my father had previously lent a gun to uncle Fausto on the farm so he could protect himself, because my uncle only had hunting weapons. So, that day my father came to pick me up, he also brought the gun back. He put it next to the driver's seat and forgot.

He stopped the car at Carlos's house and left the door open. He came in to say hello to my uncles and hurried me so we could get home:

"Let's go, let's go!"

My cousin found the gun. It was small. It looked like a toy. We were playing Western... He took the gun, pointed it at me... and took the shot!

The bullet struck the head of the femur on my left leg and then hit the passenger door on the opposite side of the car. It entered, grazed, and then exited.

I don't remember much from there. I think it bled, but no one ever told me about it. It must have been bleeding because there was a bullet entry hole in my leg and a bullet exit hole. I remember that my father took me in his arms and took off in a car to take me to the military hospital. This would be a problem for him because there had been an accident with an unregistered firearm, the weapon of a military public figure. No accident with firearms could go unnoticed at that time of the dictatorship.

But he took me, anyway. The last thing I remember is that he was distraught. As he drove at full speed to the hospital, I tried to get myself in a position where I could get extra draught from the window to breathe better. And I tried to calm him down because he was really anxious.

Emotional memory is a phenomenon that tricks us. What we remember is heavily influenced by the biases of our defense mechanisms and by the meanings our emotions ascribe to events. Antonio has his own memories.

I was in the elite Military Police special operations squad. At the time of the Revolution, we were in a state of readiness, sometimes on duty for 24 hours straight, on alert. When it was over, I wanted to run home, rest, or take Francisco to a farm to see horses, which he loved, or things like that.

"Revolution" refers to the 1964 coup d'état that initiated a military dictatorship in Brazil, which lasted until 1985.

There was this .22 caliber gun hidden in the car. And then the accident happened. Fortunately, the caliber was .22 because there would be no chance for Francisco if it was higher. The projectile pierced his thigh, but surgery was not necessary. They did everything they had to do on a medical level. And he was released.

I breathed a sigh of relief, but I was not at peace. I was left with a heavy feeling. I needed to understand where I failed. As a military man, I had to take all precautions so that no one would find the weapon, but what did I do wrong? How could the boy find the gun? It was awful and even worse for my wife at home.

Was I freezing emotionally, with Francisco?

I think I was a good provider but not an affectionate father. My wife is the one who caught my attention and fought with me. "Why don't you hug your child?" In fact, I never really hugged anyone. I had very few close relationships with anyone. For me, women were simply for sex and that was the extent of this. This was the way I was brought up.

My mother was a cabocla, a person of mixed Brazilian Indian and African descent, and my father was Polish. The home was emotionally cold, and my father was totally violent. He destroyed my brother Fausto. He beat him so hard that my mother made Fausto urinate and drink the urine to cure his internal bleeding.

48

One day, when I was 12, my father tried to catch me. Then, to defend myself, I went up and I got into a physical fight. I knew what he was like. There was no way to get out of this without facing him. I managed to escape and fled under the wooden house. We lived in Irati, in the interior of Paraná. It was a stilt house supported on pillars. He came after me, revolver in hand. I was able to protect myself behind a pillar. I, being small, was able to fit there, but he couldn´t. I stayed there until my mother, who was a teacher, came home from work to calm everything down. Later that week, she sent me to my uncle´s house in Araúcaria to escape my father. I was never to return.

The gunshot was Francisco's initiation into the world of trauma—and pain.

The trauma was collective. My cousin who, as a child, started to have several problems with drugs, and as an adult he became a totally nonfunctioning person, even experiencing mental illness. I tried to converse with him about the incident, but I never found it possible as an adult. He was visibly unbalanced.

It was an extreme trauma for my father and mother too. When I tried to find out more about what happened, the only response I got was... "It was nothing. It was just a boy thing. It was your fault. You were messing with what you shouldn't."

That was the mentality around trauma at the time. A total lack of sensitivity. But I went to school in that car every day. It was never fixed. The bullet hole was there forever, in the bodywork...

Like the others, I also forgot what they tried to erase from memory. I lost memory of an entire part of my childhood, leaving me with only flashes.

Even now, my memory of my childhood only goes back to the age of 10 or 11. There is a void from six to 10. The memory I do have is one of a body already in a lot of pain—leg pain, back pain. And I didn't know why.

The phenomenon of trauma is very complex when you are growing up. Because it hurts not just the integrity of the body, but the integrity of the developing body. It is a mind in formation, an emotional system in formation, a body in formation.

As a teenager, when I would play sports, I realized there was a crisis of some kind. Actually, I excelled in swimming, fencing, middle-distance athletic races, and other activities that I enjoyed. However, I reached a point where my thoughts and emotions overwhelmed me, leading to physical limitations that hindered my performance.

I was overwhelmed by pain. Disabling pain. I would have pain in my legs, in my back, the hips, and all that surrounds.

I've always been into individual sports, never team sports. I tried to play soccer, but I didn't know why I had zero ability to play soccer. I didn't understand that I had a hip issue, and subsequently an absence of coordination.

I didn't understand what I understand today with my work. Trauma severs parts of the neural connection in a very symbolic way. Because I didn't have a conscious memory of the accident, I also wasn't aware there was something dysfunctional about my hip.

I even think that the pain started before the age of 11, before sports, because when you have a child who grows up with pain, they sometimes don't have the cognition and language to express or interpret the pain. But they will typically have reactions to the painful experience nonverbally.

Looking back, I see that it was my case. Absolutely. Because I was super restless. There was a significant deficit of attention. I had severe *behavioral difficulties and enormous trouble focusing. My teachers overlooked that. I don't think there was a culture or sensitivity to it. I was simply categorized as a bad student.*

Antonio reflects on Francisco's school years:

We did not have a good salary. Despite this, I enrolled Francisco in Colégio Assunção, which was one of the best private schools. He then attended the Colégio Militar, the senior high school run by the Military Police, where he spent most of his high school years. He also took some private courses at Colégio Dom Bosco because he wanted to prepare well for the entrance exam to a college or university. At Dom Bosco however, he got into a fight with another student. The outcome? Both of them ended up being expelled.

When he was 15 years old, or around then, he fell down the stairs at home. It hurt badly, but he didn't break anything. There was no injury. Yet he was in severe pain for about three weeks. As it did not go away and they had not found anything more serious in the hospital, I took him to a masseuse, who referred us to a chiropractor. We got there, and the young chiropractor adjusted him. That's it, just that. Francisco got better. I think that's when his—and my—alignment with massage and chiropractic began.

But I didn't see him with any mobility problems. I didn't even see any connection between the pain from falling on the stairs and the getting shot.

He spent his years studying, and when it came time for the entrance exam to college, his mother and I thought he would study Law. And then, he came home one day very happy:

"Wow! I passed the entrance exam!"

After passing, he had the option of studying Law or attending the Guatupê Police Academy, the training academy for officers of the Military Police of Paraná. He opted for the course at the Academy.

I became interested in sports when I entered the Colégio Militar. Extreme physical activity was part of the culture, and I identified with that. When the pain started to bother me, I focused only on fencing and swimming, which allowed me to progress further despite my hidden condition. It was kind of a safe place because I didn't need the agility and coordination of soccer, for example. There, my use of the body seemed more controlled.

But I absolutely hated studying. I saw no logic, no purpose in learning. Almost all the teachers I had were incompetent. They offered nothing that attracted or engaged me. Considered a "bad student," I felt chronically inadequate, and was also very angry all the time.

In class, I had a particular notoriety... in the practice of bullying. I always teased people. Provoking was my trademark. Even when I was beaten, I provoked...

People who were influential and served as role models for me were those peers who made me feel more comfortable not wanting to study. Only gradually did I realize that they too had problems, much more than me. It's possible that some of my challenges were due to dyslexia or something of that nature.

Outside of school, my uncle Fausto was a great influence. He was a very strong figure but very tormented. His torment fascinated me, his alcoholism in particular drawing my attention. It was also very interesting to me to live in nature, as he did. The freedom he had living in the countryside, the hunting he loved to do, and the days and days he was alone in the woods were very appealing to me.

It was common for me to spend the entire school holidays with him. In November, I went to the farm in Tijucas do Sul, about 60 kilometers [37.5 miles] from Curitiba. And I would only return at

Carnaval, in February or March the following year. It was a time only of presence. No members of my family had any ability for dialogue.

Being on his farm has always been one of the best things that has happened to me. There was violence there. I had to kill animals with my own hands… everything involved a lot of violence…

But it had a very visceral nature at the same time. There was a very marked feeling of freedom and being very present. The simplicity of that life carried a kind of raw genius that left me mesmerized!

When I was there, I didn't want to live in the city anymore. I wanted that life of freedom, 100% freedom. I even imagined getting a livelihood that would allow me to have that life after college.

The scenes that filled my imagination during those seasons in the countryside—or that I witnessed firsthand—resembled the world depicted in the works of Brazilian artist Poty Lazzarotto: wooden wagons reminiscent of European immigrants, horses, and bar arguments, with bottles of wine crashing to the ground and someone with a knife in his hands.

I also interacted with my maternal grandparents, Francisco and Maria. My grandfather, Francisco, was very Polish, and my grandmother, was almost black. Francisco loved soccer and listened to the games on the radio. I knew the lineup of Brazilian teams and some national teams by heart. I remember their fervent Catholic devotion and the super-sharp knives in their kitchen.

Although I didn't exactly like to study, four teachers enchanted me with their didactic way of presenting content. Two of them were professors at the Colégio Militar. These two people were polar opposite to each other, but both were brilliant in their ability to convey content. So, the assimilation was pleasurable when the content was presented in an attractive way.

The two other teachers... they were at home!

I saw my father preparing classes for his special courses; they were brilliantly well-prepared. It was like an exercise in almost a theatrical presentation. I saw the classes he prepared on Saturday mornings, I saw his dedication, and I saw the effort embedded in the preparation of the class. And the students' enchantment was clear. His students also got the best approval ratings in the competitions in which they participated. My mother, a teacher in conventional public education, was also careful in preparing classes. Organized, methodical.

I didn't know it then, but I was falling in love with the art of teaching. I was falling in love with well-prepared classes and the way engaging teachers could effectively deliver content into the minds of students.

When it was time for the university entrance exam, I went because everyone else was doing it. But there weren't many attractive options for me. I think I thought about Law because my mother had a degree in the subject, although she never practiced as a lawyer. She also had a degree in Geography and History and several other university degrees. But none of that made sense to me.

I did well and I passed the entrance exam. I chose the Military Academy, although I'm not sure why. My father didn't want me to pursue a military career, and my mother was even less supportive.

When I entered, even I thought it was a completely illogical decision. Despite the difficulties I had at school, my mind was very sharp—I could always reason and understand things extremely quickly.

So, at the age of 17 I entered the Academy and spent two years there. But over time the feeling that it wasn't right for me grew. Then one day I came home and said,

"I'm not going anymore!"

My friends were sure that this was not for me. Everyone saw that there was an completely unsuitable path for me. Some people said,

"I don't know how you were there... None of that was for you."

My father never wanted me there anyway, and never thought the police would be an excellent career for me. My mother reacted a little with fear and insecurity about my future, that I wouldn't get a job, and so on. Neither of them had been supportive of the idea of the Academy.

But when I left the Academy, and they saw that I had no plans to enter another college, they freaked out! But I knew there was nothing in college that I wanted to do. If I had wanted to study medicine or physiotherapy, I would have become a product of the medical thinking of the time.

But that was not what I wanted. I wanted something that didn't exist yet, that still needed to be created. I wanted to have something that no one else had to offer. And I didn't really know what that was yet.

What I did know was, what I didn't want for myself. I knew that I wanted to have the ability to think for myself. Two years of taking courses at the Academy had made it clear to me that thinking independently requires particular conditions. And society, as reflected in institutions like college, exerts a powerful influence in shaping how we think. That's not what I wanted.

How was I dealing with pain during that time?

I was doing massages sporadically in the same neighborhood. I lived in the Uberaba neighborhood at that time. Those who drive from downtown Curitiba to the airport pass through it. I sometimes had chiropractic sessions but did not do physiotherapy.

I went to several orthopedists who were unimpressive and failed to present a solution. They didn't understand. You might find it unbelievable, but none of these guys ever asked for an exam, an X-ray, or a CT scan. I still didn't know that there was a link between the trauma of the gunshot and the pain I felt.

But even before dropping out of the Military Academy, I had discovered yoga. Two main experiences led me to yoga.

I must have been 15 years old. I was already studying at the Colégio Militar. One day, I went to the cinema in downtown Curitiba to watch a movie. I don't remember why I wanted to watch it. It was The Midnight Sun, a 1985 classic featuring Mikhail Baryshnikov, the famous Latvian dancer and choreographer, who is considered one of the greatest in history.

In the opening of the film, he does a solo. It was the first time I saw a male body with movement, flexibility, and strength. The scene impacted me and shocked me. From my limited and painful reality, this seemed like an incredible thing to me. I don't remember anything else from the film. I only remember his solo dance performance. And this immediately came to represent freedom to me—freedom of the body, freedom of movement.

The second experience happened a while later. I was leaving a fencing training session out of the Colégio Militar, to go to where I would take the bus home, when I stopped by chance at a newsstand on the way. There I saw Planeta magazine. Planeta was this famous trade publication on esotericism, meditation, and alternative culture more generally. The special edition at the newsstand was a yoga compendium.

I had never heard of yoga, but that magazine caught my attention. I bought a copy and opened the magazine. Instantaneously the memory of Baryshnikov's solo performance from the film resurfaced in my mind. In that moment I associated the word "freedom," which I had linked to the scene in the film, with the word "yoga."

I left there with certainty and a goal: I had to find a school to start practicing yoga. Immediately.

4

The Dark Side of The Force

To call it "love at first sight" might sound like a cliché. Describing it as "raging passion" could feel like an overstatement, as if this writer is exaggerating the narrative dose. "Enchantment" is perhaps a more fitting word.

Whatever term you or I would choose, the reality is that young Francisco felt an immense youthful enthusiasm for what was offered at a yoga school he found in downtown Curitiba. This school was run by a couple of teachers. The school, in addition to yoga, offered a massage course, which Francisco also quickly enrolled in. He saw it as a bonus that could help him combat the pain that was troubling him.

Before I first heard the word yoga, I didn't know what to do of my life. Nothing really enchanted me, nothing interested me. But when I heard that word, it was as if lightning had struck me—a very striking change. The word came to me with a certainty. It already had a defined energy. Yoga would be my professional destiny.

When I started taking classes at the school, I immediately identified what attracted me to yoga. Some people are attracted to yoga's esoteric, spiritual side, and others are attracted to the physical, bodily aspects. I identified all these things in yoga, but even then, I was already searching for something hidden in the middle of all this. I was looking for its essence.

It was a process of peeling back layer after layer until I was left with only the essence. This is precisely what I do today. I do not deprive yoga of its less tangible aspect, but I understand it and translate it in an efficient and very palpable way. And so, I deliver more to my students from the subtle side of yoga without any mysticism in my speech. In doing so, I give more than I would if I talked about chakras.

This understanding has emerged very clearly over time. But my sense that this would be the magnetic north of my path was always there from the beginning.

Young Francisco had found his direction in life, even if he couldn't yet verbalize it clearly and logically to his parents. They were both teachers with a Cartesian mentality, products of the prevailing educational paradigms in Brazilian society at the time. Antonio, as you already know, besides being a military police officer, was also a physics and mathematics professor. Lucy was a lawyer and but also a professor of history, geography, and philosophy.

I came home excited to talk about the yoga school I had found. I wanted to take classes in massage and yoga, and I needed their support to cover my course fees.

My mother did not react well, and my father didn't either. So, I had to keep at them, talking their ear off, driving them both crazy because I needed to get into those courses. My mother had a breakdown. She thought I was gay or that I would become gay... such was the homophobia that existed at home. Despite being a cultured woman, she showed this prejudiced side of her, which also came a lot from her Catholic upbringing. And she didn't hold her tongue, expressing her thoughts openly... She really thought yoga was a queer thing.

And my father, his fear? Because of his military mentality and because he knew nothing about yoga, his fear was that I would become a Hare Krishna.

From the 1960s onwards, the Hare Krishna Movement expanded rapidly from India to the West. This was partly because of the countercultural youth revolution in the United States and Europe, plus the outpouring of sympathy from show-business celebrities such as George Harrison of The Beatles, who devotedly recorded and dedicated an entire album to the times, including the hit *My Sweet Lord* that contained the famous Hare Krishna super mantra. The streets of metropolises of many countries, Brazil included, would soon be populated by cheerful groups of young mantra singers, wearing white, saffron, or orange colored dhoti pants, baggy kurtas, and saris, their faces decorated with a "tilaka" (a vertical line made of clay) without any shyness.

The youth of that era, disillusioned with mainstream society, found themselves drawn to the principles of the Hare Krishna movement. These principles emphasized devotion to God, a lacto-vegetarian diet, abstinence from alcohol and drugs, an implicit ecological ethos, sexual restraint within marriage, the cultivation of peace, and the promise of a secure path to enlightenment. In this way, the movement appealed to a generation seeking an alternative to both the dominant conservative mainstream and the radical factions advocating societal transformation through armed revolution.

One way the Hare Krishna Movement gained broader acceptance was through the establishment of restaurants that carved out a niche in the alternative gastronomic market. These eateries became known for their simple yet healthy and delicious lacto-vegetarian cuisine. The Movement's most significant annual public festival, Ratha-Yatra, eventually attracted large crowds across North America and expanded to cities in Brazil such as Rio de Janeiro, São Paulo, Belo Horizonte, Porto Alegre, Curitiba, and more. The largest rural community of the Movement in South America was established in Pindamonhangaba, in the interior of São Paulo, which followed the Movement's typical model of residential ecovillages.

Francisco would have potentially joined the Hare Krishna Movement if the young devotees had actively practiced yoga and meditation. However, this wasn't the case. Still, he sympathized with their ideals and respected their efforts to transform individuals and the world during that time. So, Antonio, had nothing to worry about—but he didn't know that.

He knew nothing about yoga. And what he learned about the Hare Krishna Movement was superficial, reflecting society's shallow perception. But I understood him—his life story and the many emotional imprints he carried. These imprints were like a powerful emotional limiter, one he would only overcome in his eighties, becoming more flexible and open than ever before.

How did his emotional limitations affect me?

Despite this issue of not expressing emotion in words and gestures, my father was a father who rolled around on the floor with the children, who was much loved by my friends in the neighborhood, and who even played when there were other children at home. I have this very clear emotional memory. In that sense, he was a fantastic father, very present. He was in a very good mood and generally at ease with life. The distance between us appeared when I reached adolescence.

My father was a man who always studied a lot. When he went to the United States for work, he explored many other things, especially in the field of health. There was always health magazines scattered throughout the house. He was a very dedicated professional, you know? The kind of people we call here "Caxias" and "CDF" [which refers to someone who is very disciplined, an "iron-head", or a nerd]. He exercised some authority as a prominent personality in his field.

He had some interesting habits. Almost every week, he would shop for groceries on the way home. He enjoyed going to the market on Saturday mornings, it was one of his favorite activities. He would carefully choose what he wanted to buy and did so with great pleasure. On Sundays, he loved cooking at home for us. He always put a lot of effort and care into everything he did.

He was a caregiver father, you know?

When I attended the Colégio Militar, it was too far from home to commute. He would wake up very early, day after day, even on the typical chilly Curitiba mornings. He always prepared breakfast for me, including a steak and eggs. It was a hearty meal, a healthy American cultural influence he had brought home from his North American days. Then, he would drive me to school. This happened every single day throughout my high school years.

FRANCISCO KAIUT with EDVALDO PEREIRA LIMA

I also admired his values and habits. At least twice a week, he went out with his tennis shoes to run and practice his sport. He was very consistent.

When our estrangement began in my adolescence, I could see more clearly that my father was very lonely. He never had friends. He had colleagues in the barracks, but no friends. Nobody visited us at home, and he did not visit anyone's house.

He never wasted time with any distractions. I never saw him standing in front of a television. He was always reading or working, filling his inner universe with strong interests. The amount he read was inspiring to me. And he always gave me absolute freedom to read whatever I wanted.

Looking back long after adolescence, I realized that he, as a man, had a lot of difficulty connecting with his son. I had trouble sustaining a dialogue that wasn't childish, playful, or filled with provocation and silly things. Therefore, we couldn't transition properly—from me being a child to a teenager and then to an adult, and from him being the father of a child to the father of a teenager and ultimately to the father of a man.

But that was his way, so he went, so he was.

As a writer, biographer, and archaeologist of the soul—not just of the material facts of life stories—I need to provoke and explore with tact during this delicate moment of revealing and unveiling.

What about Francisco's mother? And what legacy did each of them leave him?

Unlike my father, who took great pleasure in what he did, I didn't know if my mother enjoyed what she did. However, both had the characteristic of preparing and planning high-quality classes.

My mother was a great companion. Although she was a very conflicted person, our relationship was good. There was no emotional distance with her.

There was, instead, a distancing due to other circumstances during my adolescence. Both my father and mother worked hard; he did so because he enjoyed it, and she because being a teacher involved a high volume of work, which was usual for her. Both worked three shifts, leaving us with very little contact time. They loved taking road trips through the interior of Brazil during vacations, which I hated. I preferred to stay at home or at my uncle's farm, where I loved immersing myself in Nature, in absolute freedom.

My mother was a brilliant, super-intellectual woman, but her emotional intelligence was nearly non-existent. She possessed a rational intellect with a deeply emotional soul, yet this didn't manifest as emotional intelligence, if that makes sense.

Despite her strong intellectual abilities, she was often overwhelmed by very basic and very negative emotions, specifically pessimism, depression, and frustration. Very negative. Additionally, she was the daughter of a deeply Catholic Polish couple and was raised in a very conservative Catholic environment in the outback of the neighboring state of Santa Catarina.

So, she came from a very dark place, which was taboo for her to talk about—a place marked by significant violence and the harsh repression of Catholicism. She struggled with various issues related to her body, health, obesity, and smoking. By the time she reached her 50s, she described herself as old and harbored a dream of retiring and doing nothing else. Tragically, she passed away very young, at the age of 54, from a very aggressive disease that began as bowel cancer. In a way, it seemed like a self-fulfilling prophecy, you know?

Her prominent Caucasian features complemented her physical profile of short hair and stature of one meter and sixty centimeters [5'3"] In her challenges with obesity, she at one point weighed over a hundred kilos [220 lbs]. Through a rigorous regimen, she successfully halved her weight, but the inner conflict persisted. It wasn't just about weight, but also her relationship with food. Unfortunately, she never found a place of pleasure with things that were actually good for her.

Before the disease, she liked to dress well. She had all the classic feminine vanities. But with the disease, she became sloppy in general. It seems that the ghosts took over, like a chronicle of a death foretold.

Antonio:

Lucy was very strict and demanding. Everything with her had to be perfect. But I understood her, being a teacher, a school principal, everything had to be correct, you know? But there was no conflict between me and her because of Francisco. Sometimes, I just said that I didn't agree with some attitudes she took with him, but I understood her standard of demand.

She was emotionally distant, but a good mother by caring for him in her own way. She was doing very well in what she understood was her duty. The duty of care as a mother.

I was more relaxed with Francisco's things. Lucy, a typical native of Santa Catarina, enjoyed dishes like carreteiro rice, missionary chicken, and tropeiro beans. I, on the other hand, had a penchant for some unconventional gaúcho foods. Lucy had a deep appreciation for gaúcho music, and we often frequented dancing restaurants in Porto Alegre, where we would enjoy live performances by singers she admired, such as the Argentine naturalized Brazilian, Dante Ramón Ledezma.

Gaúcho refers to the people from the southern state of Rio Grande do Sul, and to all things related to its culture.

Despite my lack of enthusiasm for dancing, I joined her on the dance floor to make her happy. We continued to include Francisco in our outings until he turned 14 years old. And then one day, he said: "Oh, father, I can't stand these trips with you anymore."

And that was okay with me. Francisco did not travel with us anymore.

When he first mentioned the yoga school, I found it rather peculiar. I assumed he might have been influenced by the Hare Krishna group, people with earrings, ponytails, skirts, and sometimes shaved heads. It wasn't a matter of prejudice, simply an unfamiliarity with a world that seemed odd to me. I even speculated about the presence of drugs.

However, as I realized that he wanted to do it very badly, and his mother didn't want it at all, I really got involved. I told her:

"The boy really wants to do it. Let him do it, all right?"

She stayed reluctant, so I proposed:

"Let's make a deal. The massage course is held on weekends. Since I have weekends off, I'll attend the course with Francisco!"

And so, we embarked on the journey together. We studied massage, practiced on each other, and successfully completed the course.

When we finished the massage course, he wanted to stay in school. This time to take the yoga course. As I had already seen there was nothing strange there—that it was not a drug trafficking point—I just said:

"Ok! Take the course!"

Antonio could not have known that this would not only be an introduction to yoga for his son, but also the indirect beginning of his own journey in the world of yoga, leading to a great transformation in his life and the start of a path that would intersect with Francisco's at various points.

What yoga did Francisco learn at this school?

The "beans and rice" of conventional yoga, as he recalls. A lot of hatha yoga, the traditional approach to working with the body and the classic postures, the asanas.

The school also offered a more sophisticated and ambitious form of practice, vidya yoga, which promised self-knowledge and personal growth, ultimately leading the practitioner to full awakening of consciousness at a spiritual level and beyond.

Young Francisco found both the yoga and massages courses to be very good, as well as the teachers who led them. And thus, perhaps dazzled by what he found, he did not filter or critically think about teaching method and model of knowledge transmission that vidya yoga adopted. It involved the traditional Hindu approach, rooted in a close guru-disciple relationship, which required a level of surrender and submission that is unfamiliar and often uncomfortable for those in Western culture.

What, then, was the state of yoga teaching and practice in Brazil during Francisco's initial foray into this field? What historical developments had unfolded to create the conditions that allowed him to encounter a gateway to his path—one situated so close to his hometown?

It is said that the long journey of yoga—from its origins in India to the southern cone of America and its touchdown in Brazil—began at the end of the nineteenth century through newspaper reports. These reports introduced the word "yoga" to the public for the first time. They served as a gateway of ideas, planting into the collective consciousness the first inklings that something different existed in the East, drawing attention to possibilities for unimaginable achievements that could be within our reach. The articles told stories about Indian fakirs (holy men), who, through this strange practice called yoga, could have nails driven into their tongues and be imprisoned in a cave without water and food and come out alive 30 days later as if nothing much had happened.

The second phase of the gradual and informal awareness among Brazilians regarding yoga occurred in the first two decades of the twentieth century. This observation comes from a meticulous study on the history of yoga in Brazil, conducted with the scholarly rigor expected of a prestigious academic institution. The article titled Beginnings of yoga in Brazil, c.1910-1920, was in the journal *Movimento*, published by the Federal University of Rio Grande do Sul's physical education department.

Authors Andrea Calazans Rocha Dias and Cleber Dias highlight that this period marked a significant shift in how yoga was perceived in Brazil. It was a time characterized by the dissemination of Portuguese-translated books, newspaper articles, and conferences, which began to distance yoga from its earlier portrayal as something exotic or folkloric. These efforts were largely spearheaded by organizations with mystical and spiritual orientations.

The champion of this endeavor was the Theosophical Society, which was founded in New York by the renowned Russian esoteric leader Helena Petrovna Blavatsky and prominent American lawyer and journalist Colonel Henry Steel Olcott around 1875. By the turn of the century, the Society had established stores and study groups in Brazil, culminating in the creation of a national section. This exponentially expanded the discourse on yoga, shifting it from being an object of sensationalist curiosity to being appreciated for the spiritual richness of its philosophy and the scientifically recognized health benefits of its practice.

The earliest public display of yoga practice in Brazil is believed to have occurred in 1928, initiated by the Brazilian section of the Society. They invited the Ceylonese (modern day Sri Lanka) master Curuppumullage Jinarajadasa to Rio de Janeiro and São Paulo. Press reports of the time stated that Jinarajadasa's lectures and presentations captured the attention of a "colossal audience" and received "prolonged applause". In the wake of the Theosophical Society's initiatives, other spiritualistic groups also contributed to embedding yoga into Brazil's collective cultural landscape, organizing further events.

Yoga truly started to become popular in Brazil in the 1940s, following a period of complex cultural exchange that included influences from India, France, and Uruguay. According to one historical account, French practitioners who were aligned with traditional Indian methods chose to move the focus of their teaching and practice to South America, given they were disheartened by the ravages of World War I and sensed the ominous approach of World War II.

One such pioneer was the individual known, by his initiatory name, as Swami Asuri Kapila. He set up a center in Montevideo, the capital of Uruguay, where he trained yoga teachers for the South American continent and promoted the practice. It is believed that this teacher made a significant impression in Porto Alegre in 1944. He also likely sent one of his disciples, Swami Sevananda (the Frenchman Léo Costet de Mascheville) to present at an important congress in Rio de Janeiro in 1947. The event was striking enough to draw an estimated audience of five thousand people. There is some historical disagreement regarding the relationship between Kapila and Sevananda, with some sources, which may not be reliable, suggesting that Sevananda was in fact Kapila's teacher.

Sevananda returned to Brazil in 1952, embarking on a mission to spread yoga. In 1953, he traveled throughout the country and eventually settled in Resende, located within the state of Rio de Janeiro. There, he established a monastery and a mystical association, both of which are regarded as the first dedicated spaces for yoga practice in Brazil.

Over four decades, lectures, conferences, publications, and visits by foreign masters cultivated a fertile ground for yoga in Brazil. By the 1950s, the practice had definitively gained popularity, marked by the emergence of Brazilian teachers who adapted and presented yoga in a format more accessible to the local population. This period also saw the first publications of specialized works by Brazilian authors.

As Sevananda persisted in training new generations of teachers, notable figures began to emerge in the field of yoga. Among them was military officer Caio Miranda who, inspired by a lecture given by the French master in 1947, went on to have an illustrious pioneering career in yoga. Another significant contributor was José Hermógenes, also an army officer, who turned to yoga as a complementary therapy for tuberculosis. Following his recovery, he dedicated his life to teaching and writing about the therapeutic benefits of yoga.

Throughout the 1960s, both men became esteemed yoga teachers in Rio de Janeiro, alongside Luiz Sérgio Alvarez De Rose. Professors Hermógenes and De Rose, in particular, established themselves as prominent figures in the yoga community, each creating a distinct brand and network of yoga practices characterized by their unique styles.

Less famous but no less pioneering, the judoka Shotaro Shimada also played a significant role in advancing yoga. At the end of the 1950s, he began training teachers in São Paulo. One of his students, Maria Celeste de Castilho, was instrumental in introducing yoga into the exclusive circles of the city's Jockey Club. By the early 1970s, at the time Francisco was born, another of Shimada's disciples, Maria Helena de Barros Freire, had initiated the first university program designed to train yoga teachers.

Francisco's potential place in the history of yoga is set against the backdrop of this dynamic reality. The path he would follow had been laid by the dedicated service and groundwork of those who came before him in the yoga community.

And then, fired by the rocket of youthful enthusiasm, he launches himself into the eye of the hurricane.

I was around 17 or 18 years old when the yoga school where I was taking studying and practicing was put up for sale. I took a piece of land that my father had given me as a gift, on Guaratuba beach, on the coast of Paraná, and sold it. With the money, I bought the school. It was all set up in a commercial building in downtown Curitiba, with 60 or 70 students enrolled.

I started teaching on my own and worked hard. I always enjoyed working a lot, and I soon discovered that teaching yoga was very pleasurable for me. Then the school boomed. I taught the same course that I had studied, and before I knew it, I had over a hundred students!

So, I was absolutely certain that my place was in the classroom! The students were well-suited to the practice—executives, bank employees, and people who worked in telecommunications companies.

I realized that I had a knack for translating situations in a way that made sense to every new student who arrived.

I don't know if it was due to my parents' influence, but I started preparing my classes thoroughly. I was never unprepared and never repetitive. The classes went excellently. I always considered both the individual and the collective aspects. I crafted lesson plans that combined individual needs into a cohesive, collective experience.

It was also exciting to see that people assumed I enjoyed teaching yoga because it helped them feel better. Many came with lower back, neck, and knee pain, seeking relief. It was fascinating to see how many people like that showed up.

Everything seemed to be going very well, or so I thought. However, I was unaware of the administrative side of things. I had no experience in management. My father, being a civil servant, couldn't prepare me for this since he knew nothing about it either. I trusted the couple who previously owned the school deeply, having a very close, almost guru-disciple type of relationship with them.

Then they noticed my growing success and put the idea in my head that I had to move to a bigger location to accommodate more students. I believed them and made the change. However, they didn't prepare me for the challenges that came with it. The existing students didn't follow me to the new location, and I couldn't attract new ones. I burned through all my savings and had to close the school.

That's when I realized that the people who had sold me the school were good teachers, but they weren't very honest. They engaged in some questionable activities. They manipulated the percentage I paid them for using their courses, as if it were a license. They also controlled the flow of money, lacked transparency, mishandled expenses, and failed to provide the guidance I needed.

They were not bad people, but they had character flaws. Although the courses were excellent, they had a tendency to skim money. They recommended an accountant and a lawyer to help me, but both turned out to be somewhat dishonest. There were instances of money theft and situations where they claimed to be short on cash and asked me for advances on payments. I couldn't escape these issues.

They had sold me the school, and I had paid, so you might think they no longer had any involvement or rights in the business. However, these so-called gurus still tried to maintain control and directly interfere.

After I closed the school, I moved away from home, and from my father.

Those teachers had decided to launch a new project in a small town in the metropolitan region of Curitiba. They bought a piece of land and opened an ashram there, a kind of free yoga university. But they didn't have any infrastructure, they didn't have the conditions for it. It was a misguided venture from the beginning.

But there I was, living in the ashram and working for them, teaching there and in other places for them. It took me a while to realize that I was in a situation of heavy manipulation. And it wasn't just material. It hurt me spiritually too.

However, I needed this close interaction to make it very clear to me that they were not, in fact, honest people.

It's like... you know that series of classic science fiction movies, Star Wars? Jedi warriors had to learn to use the energy of the force, the light side of it. But they could not be naïve. They had to learn that the dark side also exists. And they had to learn how to not let it dominate them. They couldn't let anger consumer them. Otherwise, they would cross over to the dark side of the force. And they would be lost.

Eventually, I knew I had to break free. I knew I had to cut ties completely, even if it meant getting my heartbroken concerning yoga. Even if the price to pay was embracing a new pain.

5

Writing Right through Crooked Lines

When we join mythology with Jung's archetypes, as we saw in chapter one, stories gain perspective, and discovering their meaning becomes even more pleasurable, whether it be real-life stories like Francisco's or fictional ones like the film he recalled a moment ago.

The marriage between these two forms of knowledge of mythology and archetypes is best consecrated when the storyteller—in cinema or in this book—employs the resource of the Hero's Journey. The Journey represents the processes of our existence, and the hero, or heroine, is each one of us. Such an underlying theme of Francisco's life was implicitly hinted at in his reference to *Star Wars*.

Certainly, Francisco encountered the dark side of the world, in both people and things. This growth in awareness from one of youthful innocence and naivety to the adult discovery that reality is not pure or monochrome, is not easy. The positive and the negative are part of the Nature of things. But if the blow of this encounter with the dark side is too strong, the hero falls on the Journey, and lands in vulnerable situation in which he needs "internal rescue." The paradox of this term is that the hero's inner efforts to help himself are insufficient to escape the jam. He also needs external help.

Would it be Antonio who would help?

I had a lot of conflict with Francisco when he got more and more involved with the couple from the yoga school and ashram. He started to spend a great deal of time there and a great distance came between us when he went to live in the ashram.

It was very strange when I realized that they were indoctrinating the people who were there. One of the things they said is that the yogin, the yoga practitioner, cannot value father and mother. This idea of family antagonism got Francisco. It was as if he had found a new home. I was very worried.

The distance between us grew primarily because Francisco cherished the freedom of immersing himself in yoga throughout the entire day when he began teaching. This enjoyment sustained him, even as challenges arose. His passion for yoga, especially teaching in the classroom, served as an antidote to the toxicity of his uncomfortable relationship with that couple.

The distance would last a long time however, even when Francisco came to his senses, realizing that he would definitely need to break the vicious circle created through dependence, he did so by his own decision. He moved away from the ashram, from that environment that had become too unhealthy for his soul. More than anything, it was an act of spiritual liberation.

But he did not return home. He distanced himself from yoga. Somewhat lost in his life direction, he plunged into pain. In the search for a cure for what bothered him concretely, in the physical. Without finding relief or explanation that would satisfy. This perhaps, revealed the other pain that he threw into the unconscious, that of disappointment in those he trusted; the disillusionment of finding his own limitations in the practical, organizational side of things and the need for a dream to be resolved in the material world, to be fulfilled.

I entered a phase of a lot of anguish... depression... melancholy... even sadness. It was not a phase of feeling that life was unfair. It was a phase of feeling really depressed, with a lot of physical pain. I felt drained of energy... It felt like my body was completely locked up and stuck, which was also keeping my head all bound up too.

It was a clear situation where rescue was needed. Help would come. But in due time. The time of destiny is not that of our ego, nor is it always written with certainty.

Antonio:

As you already know, I had decided to accompany Francisco and learn massage. Yoga concepts were also included in that course. I learnt that in addition to the physical body, we have the etheric, emotional, and mental bodies. And we have chakras. The teachers kept encouraging us,

"We will feel the chakra..."

The students would look for the chakra, but I didn't feel anything...

Of course, I came from classical science. I was a physics and mathematics teacher. I couldn't conceive of anything that wasn't material or physical and that I couldn't measure or weigh. But I was intrigued,

"What are these guys talking about?"

One day, I saw a brochure from a chiropractic professional—the same professional to whom I had taken Francisco once for a treatment session. This time, I wanted to know more about chiropractic. I read that one of its principles is that when there is a blockage in the spine, for example, in a vertebra, it involves an interruption of the flow of energy to the area.

I was very intrigued by that, too. What is this energy? Does it really exist? Because I didn't feel any of that. If it existed, I wanted to know it!

So, I went to take a chiropractic course, a real training, with Dr. Matheus de Souza in São Paulo. It was about three and a half years of training, on weekends.

I was motivated, first, due to intellectual curiosity. The curiosity to know. What is this energy that these people talk about, that I don't feel? And then, secondly, I had an experience where I saw a result of something apparently esoteric when working on a family member, that showed me there is something real there, even if I don't understand it. Because it produced an effect.

I had already taken the massage course and the chiropractic course when a relative of my wife came to visit us at home one day. He arrived dragging a leg, in great pain. He asked,

"Help me, I don't know what else to do."

I applied a technique to find where his body may be blocked. We don't put our hands on the person. The hand stays at a distance. I applied the technique as he lay on his back, not seeing what I was doing.

After a few minutes, he said,

"Antonio, my leg has frozen."

I thought, he doesn't know what I'm doing, I didn't touch him, but his leg froze. Why? Then I realized that although I didn't feel it, a field existed. The frozen leg was a field.

So, I did the Lasègue Test on him. It was positive. I told him,

"Go see a doctor, go for an exam. Because you have a herniated disc."

I realized that I had touched his field, which revealed a mechanical blockage. The chiropractic test confirmed that he had this herniated disc. But he didn't want to go to the doctor.

However, about four months later, he called me,

"I'm leaving the hospital. I just had an exam. I have a herniated disc!"

I began to associate one thing with the other to understand about this energy.

So that you and I understand what Antonio is saying, allow me to define the word "field" as it is used in this narrative. This definition will be very useful throughout the book. I draw on a definition given by American physician Bruce Lipton, a leading researcher in epigenetics, a revolutionary area of biological science. I have lightly edited his definition for clarity, while respecting its essence: *A field is a set of invisible forces in motion that influence and affect visible reality.*

Does it make sense to you?

It was finally making sense to Antonio. As it made sense for Antonio to apply the Lasègue Test, a physical examination that can detect if there is nerve root irritation in the lower spine, so he could determine whether his relative's pain and inability to take his morning walk was hindered due to a herniated disc.

It also made a lot of sense for Antonio to sacrifice his weekends to study at the Brazilian Institute of Chiropractic, the organization founded by the most famous name in this health practice in the country, Manoel Matheus de Souza.

Chiropractic, also referenced as spinal or joint manipulation, is a non-invasive, non-pharmaceutical modality in the health field. The therapist uses their hands to treat issues involving the spine and its effects on the nervous system—that is, it looks to address not only the physical body but also subtle, energetic patterns.

It was developed in the United States at the end of the nineteenth century, eventually arriving in Brazil with the help of

North American professionals. According to an informal historical chronicle by Carlos Braghini Júnior, the first chiropractic training course in Brazil took place in Curitiba in 1958. However, it was closed in 1964 due to possible pressure from conventional medical associations and the persecution of professionals by the military dictatorship that came into power that year.

One of the course graduates, Manoel Matheus de Souza, took the lead in defending the professionals and renewing their practice, adapting it to Brazilian conditions. He eventually created a protocol and method that bears his name.

But Matheus paid a very high price for his boldness. Forced to leave Curitiba, he was imprisoned by the military regime at least once. Despite this, his combative spirit persisted as he continued to provide clinical care, teach, and propagate chiropractic underground for many years. Consequently, his trajectory during that period is marked by frequent changes in address and practice locations, as he sought to evade persecution. Braghini notes that during this time Matheus had residences in Porto Alegre, Rio de Janeiro, Florianópolis, and Presidente Prudente, in the state of São Paulo.

By the time Antonio went to take the course in São Paulo, the situation had changed, and Brazil had returned to a democratic state. Matheus was then consolidating his reputation as the most important figure in the history of chiropractic in Brazil.

Training gave me the certainty that massage and chiropractic techniques and maneuvers were effective and could produce results, which motivated me to start working in healthcare in my spare time. During those early year, I also learned polarity therapy on my own.

Applying all this made me even more curious about this energy issue. How could such a good result, like pain relief, be achieved only with manual contact? So, as soon as I retired from the Military Police, I started working full-time as a healthcare professional. I rented space in a clinic to offer my services.

When I was already far along this path and had a full schedule, I went to São Paulo to meet Francisco, who had taken some courses there. We were very far apart, really. I found him a little dejected and discouraged. And then...

"You know that your mother and I really like to go dancing in Porto Alegre. We continue to go there once a month. But whenever I leave, my clients complain. 'Fifteen days without massage? You can't go!'"

Then I looked at him,

"Do you want to help me? I need someone to see clients on the days I am away with your mother. You are very good at massage and yoga. And I will teach you techniques from polarity therapy."

He agreed! He started working with me, and I taught him all the techniques. He grasped them like this—*snaps his fingers*—quickly! He was increasingly dedicating himself to polarity therapy, becoming very efficient in what he did. He assisted entire families, parents, and children alike. From then on, I was at ease because I could travel, and my clients were not without help. And there came a time when he had more customers than me! And that was okay.

Polarity therapy?

It is a complementary therapy developed by Randolph Stone, an Austrian-American chiropractor, osteopath, and naturopath. It integrates Western medical knowledge with principles of Eastern energy medicine found in Ayurveda and traditional Chinese practices, as well as concepts from diverse disciplines including yoga, esoteric hermetic studies, the Kabbalah, and alchemy.

Throughout his extensive career, Randolph Stone alternated working in the United States and India. He was also a pioneer of craniosacral therapy. Stone believed that the purpose of polarity therapy was to facilitate the body's natural healing processes by balancing the positive and negative poles of the energy currents that run throughout the body. The practice involves seeking this vital balance through a conscious awareness of self.

My father's post-retirement transformation has been striking, especially considering his traditional military career. He held significant posts, such as unit commander and chief of capital city policing and was even offered the position of Secretary of Public Security just as he approached retirement. He did not take it up, however. He joked with me and said he had taken up the role of Secretary of Massage instead.

When we ended up working together, a period of great professional learning and growth began, for him and for me. Sometime after retirement, he decided to complete his training, so he took a massage course in the United States.

Antonio began a course at Myotherapy Massage College in Salt Lake City, Utah. This school, established by health pioneer Jim Foster, specializes in various unique approaches to wellness. Foster's myotherapy technique specifically addresses and seeks to prevent soft tissue pain and restricted joint movement resulting from muscle dysfunction or issues with the fascia—the interconnected tissues of nerves and blood vessels surrounding muscles. Central to his method is the "triad of health," which fosters integration among the body, mind, and spirit, with emotions serving as the crucial link that unifies these elements.

The course spanned three years, combining distance learning with a compulsory annual residency at the school's main facility for hands-on training. As a reward for his dedication, Antonio was gifted with additional training in polarity therapy.

My father and I spent eight years learning together, culminating in me taking a chiropractic course in São Paulo. Throughout this period, we were united by a self-taught ethos, exchanging ideas and engaging in joint research. We immersed ourselves in the works of internationally respected authors from all around the globe in the fields of naturopathy and natural health. These experiences profoundly influenced our approaches and expanded our perspectives.

Randolph Stone emerged as the most significant influence. Other notable figures included Dr. Katsusuki Serizawa, who devised numerous massage protocols for chronic conditions, and André de Sambucy, a French rheumatologist who pioneered profound deep tissue massage techniques for chronic diseases in the 1940s. Jim Foster also left a mark with his meticulously crafted method.

But it was Matheus de Souza who stood apart as a genius. His skill was unparalleled. Though I would later experience the treatments of chiropractors, masseurs, osteopaths, and polarity therapists in the United States and England, none matched the exceptional quality of Matheus's touch.

Not only did I attend lessons with him, but I also traveled to São Paulo from time to time for personal consultations, despite the high cost for a mere 15-minute session.

During one of the very first consultations, he immediately identified my hip issue and the trauma that I still had no conscious memory of. There was a knowing. I knew I had been shot. But I hadn't yet made a conscious correlation between the gunshot and the trauma. There was no link.

When he started manipulating the area, he noted,

"There's something here."

I denied it,

"No, there's nothing."

He insisted,

"Yes, there is!"

I remained in denial,

"No, there isn't!"

"Yes, there is!"

"No, there isn't!"

"There is!"

"There isn't!"

"There is!"

"Holy shit, yes, there is! I was shot!"

Then the recollection and resurfacing of my memory truly occurred. That's when I started seeing things differently.

When pain becomes an undeniable reality, you might find yourself desperately seeking temporary relief. This pursuit can become a cycle: the more relief you chase, the more you find yourself outsourcing your pain. You move from one medication to another, from doctor to doctor, from the distress of one surgical procedure to the next. And so, the snowball grows, escalating into an ever-increasing crescendo of suffering.

However, when you continue to proactively and constructively seek solutions, but at the same time understand that accepting pain is the first step... which means to look at it... welcome it... welcome yourself and the suffering that exists... then you start to gain clarity.

You begin to realize that there is a way. There is a path that generates a solution. But it passes through the eye of pain.

Even so, the pain may not go away. However, you have an ace up your sleeve. If you accept the pain, you will live in peace with it. However, if you do not accept it, peace will not exist.

When you embrace the pain, and accept that it may be immutable, pain is no longer determinant. Almost everything that is scary lives in our imagination. So, when you look into the eye of the thing, it melts down.

So, you can consider Matheus a mentor to my father and me. He suggested many of the books and authors that we ended up exploring. We did deep research in areas where people did not dedicate themselves.

It was a very crazy thing that was happening between us, in the mutual learning and a lot of exchange. I approached things more conceptually and reflectively; my father approached them more practically. I identified a technique; he trained the technique.

It was shocking to realize that while the world was dedicated to medicine and a disease perspective, we were finding non-medical paths that were dedicated to health. We found techniques that nobody had heard of yet, such as the "vertebral percussion technique". Things like that often seemed like some technique of a Jedi warrior or Yogic Master... as they really worked and delivered results, in practice. We saw a fantastic volume of results with patients!

Antonio:

At a certain point, Francisco revealed his desire to teach yoga classes. I said okay. We became his first students—his mother and me! And then more people started arriving.

When we needed to move from the room we had rented, a woman, Fanny, a massage client who liked him very much, offered a place in a property she owned, where she had a spiritist center near the Parque Barigui neighborhood. And then, when we rented a house downtown to be a clinic of our own, his mother helped prepare the place. She no longer had any reservations about Francisco being involved with yoga.

The joint work facilitated rapprochement between my father and me. A mutual admiration gradually emerged. My admiration primarily stemmed from observing his ability to change—it was remarkable to witness his shift in values and his consistency in building a whole new career. This renewal in his life laid the foundation for open and meaningful dialogue between us.

My relationship with my mother also evolved. My mother's admiration of me came from her supporting the things that were valuable to me, an admiration tinged with friendship. During her more lucid moments, free from her emotional disturbances, we had excellent dialogues. And before she got sick, she won my admiration. Despite issues with her body, she broke free from the inertia and took steps in a surprising direction by coming to yoga!

Antonio:

The number of students was increasing. The years went by, and Francisco was working hard.

There were days when he arrived at the clinic at seven in the morning and left at eleven at night. I continued to help him. I felt that he needed to grow and free himself from the yoga and experiences with school he originally went to. He continued to learn by himself, watching video classes that emphasized classical, rigid postures. It was very aggressive yoga that pushed one beyond their limits.

I didn't like that Francisco gave so much of himself. Perhaps in wanting to accelerate his learning, he called a cousin of his, Ed Cleso, to help him. Ed was then a muscular and robust young man. He came in and pushed and pulled and did whatever was necessary to help Francisco.

When he had the idea to bring an American teacher to Brazil and get some private lessons, his mother and I supported him. We spent about 15 days taking classes with this teacher from New York, at our house on the beach in Guaratuba. The classes were for Francisco to have a better education, they were not for me. I never wanted to be a yoga teacher. I was satisfied with being a student only. My focus was different.

Later we brought in an American specialist in polarity therapy. We no longer had the house in Guaratuba, but I rented a two-story house in the same area, and we studied and practiced with this teacher for about 15 days. This time, the classes were for him and me.

I bought Yoga Journal, *the most significant yoga trade publication in the United States. I kept calling the teachers listed in the publication to find out if any of them would come to Brazil to give me private lessons. It happened that Theresa Gayle Rowland, owner of Studio Yoga, answered the phone herself. She accepted on the spot.*

Upon learning about Francisco's work, Theresa ignited the first spark of destiny that propelled the young Brazilian into the international yoga circuit. She encouraged him to attend a meeting of teachers in Italy. And invited him to teach in her studio in Madison, New Jersey, which is very close to New York City, the iconic Big Apple and arguably the most cosmopolitan global metropolis.

The doors opened to the world. By now, Francisco might have been scalded by the dual, bipolar nature of reality. Or maybe not. Indifferent to this, fate had reserved for him great discoveries. And great disappointments.

6

Three Episodes and an Extended Season: International Baptism

Born in New York and raised in the suburbs of the city in neighboring New Jersey, Theresa Gayle Rowland built a successful career as a yoga teacher. She founded her own Studio Yoga in Madison, just 30 or so miles (49 kms) from the heart of Manhattan. There, she established a respectable teacher training program. An adept of Iyengar Yoga, she frequently trained at the institute of her master, B.K.S. Iyengar, in Pune, India. Theresa also enjoyed studying with instructors from different parts of the world.

As a seasoned teacher and advocate of yoga, Theresa's international predisposition likely played a key role in her ready acceptance of an invitation from an unknown practitioner in a distant country. She had limited knowledge of Brazil and its culture, despite the heart of New Yorks' Brazilian community being only 15 miles (25 kms) from her studio in the neighboring suburb of Newark. Yet, she didn't hesitate in accepting the invitation. She could hardly have anticipated that answering a surprise phone call from a novice Brazilian teacher would lead her to visit Curitiba three times, in what would become a remarkable journey of mutual growth. As a mentor, she would open international doors for Francisco. Yet, by fate's design, she also had much to learn from the audacious apprentice who, through their intertwined destinies, became her unlikely teacher.

When Theresa came to Brazil to give me private lessons, I discovered she was a highly experienced figure deeply immersed in the international yoga scene. She brought with her an extensive arsenal of techniques and possibilities. However, I realized that an equally strong foundation of logic, concepts, and clear guidelines was necessary. I also observed that she was more interested in learning about my practices than in simply imparting her own knowledge.

Between Theresa's visits, I began experimental work in Curitiba with a small group of practitioners, exploring approaches that diverged from traditional yoga. Before long, she invited me to New York to teach my methods at her studio and to study with her.

I didn't accept it, because I was particularly interested in Theresa's other invitation: attending a major gathering of Iyengar yoga teachers in Italy.

Theresa was eager to insert me into this international yoga circle. Her school was very influential, and she was a great support of the community worldwide, actively promoting the practice globally. Every year this remarkable woman went to Italy, to teach at this event. She always took another guest teacher with her, alternating each year, sometimes it was Patricia Walden, other times John Schumacher. She also wanted me to meet and study with one of them, whoever was there, in Italy, at that time. When I got there, I knew it was Patricia's turn, a very good friend of hers.

A celebrity in the world of yoga and a prominent icon in the history of the practice in the United States, Patricia Walden is considered one of the most important figures in the list of Iyengar Yoga teachers worldwide. At a very young age, in 1976, she met B.K.S. Iyengar, immediately becoming a devoted disciple, spending long periods practicing with the master annually in Pune while he was alive. The devotion would not prevent her from crafting her own approach to practicing and teaching Iyengar Yoga. She further popularized this style of yoga through her DVDs and teacher training courses in the United States and abroad. To this day, as this text is written, she remains committed to this work, operating out of Boston and Cambridge. These cities are not only renowned for their vibrant cultural milieu, shaped by prestigious institutions like Harvard, MIT, and Northeastern, but are also place that embrace alternatives to mainstream society, such as yoga.

Patricia was instrumental in establishing Iyengar Yoga in North America through her teaching and the creation of organizations and entities associated with the B.K.S. Iyengar Institute. However, in Italy, the Iyengar lineage encountered more obstacles. Teachers such as Gabriela Giubilaro, Grazia Melloni, and other pioneers faced difficulties in solidifying the tradition within their country.

Florence, the capital of Tuscany, is an art-city famous for its numerous galleries and iconic works by the Renaissance masters such as Leonardo da Vinci, Michelangelo, and Sandro Botticelli. It also became the headquarters of the initiatives of Iyengar's Italian disciples.

It is not by chance, then, that the event Francisco would attend was in Tuscany—a region that evokes idyllic, romantic visions of undulating hills, tall cypress trees swaying in the breeze, bales of hay in the fields, and medieval towns with historic towers and narrow streets forbidden to cars, all surrounded by ancient stone walls.

Francisco would have the opportunity to enjoy this tourist setting of pleasure, indulging in gastronomic delights of Tuscan cuisine, while savoring the wines—which he enjoys—from the local cellars. But the most important experience awaiting him on his first European adventure was far from the world of Bacchus, the God of wine. It was closer to his mythological counterpart Chiron, already a companion of the emerging Brazilian teacher.

The teachers' meeting took place in the countryside, about 37 miles (60 kms) from Florence, on a farm owned by Gabriela's family in the commune of Rapolano Terme, a region famous for its thermal water spas. In Italian geopolitics, a commune is equivalent to a municipality or town in other nations. Rapolano is one of the thirty-six communes that make up the province of Siena; with Siena one of ten provinces that make up the region of Tuscany. Italy has twenty regions, of which Tuscany is one of the best known.

The region is wonderful, with a phenomenal view between Florence and Siena. The classroom was actually a giant shed, very beautiful. Participants were hosted throughout the region, some at the event site itself. An Italian cook prepared fantastic Mediterranean food. And, of course, it was a big, lucrative event, with people from all over the world and a lot of money.

The event was very interesting, and it was nice to be there and interact with so many people devoted to yoga. I ended up studying with Patricia and establishing contact with John, with whom I would exchange a lot of emails from then on, talking a lot about my doubts and questions.

But what did I see of yoga?

I saw work that did not enchant me. It was work that was crude and aggressive. Clearly, it was not sustainable. And I saw people who appeared unbalanced, depressed, anxious, with dysregulated nervous systems—yoga teachers!

Basically, my first exposure to Iyengar Yoga gave me a big scare! Because I expected to find the results that Iyengar himself obtained, and I did not. However, this experience proved to be a crucial lesson. I needed to find my own way. I needed to find yoga itself and not get caught in names and prevailing trends. I was left with this internal conviction that I should not let anyone else contaminate my work and that I should no longer take any course with anyone in yoga except Theresa.

This experience deeply solidified my commitment to free-thinking—a value I hold above all else. It was also the first time I discovered, to my surprise, my ability to keenly observe and identify patterns in people's bodies. I noticed several recurring issues, even among yoga teachers, that seemed to predispose them to future problems.

A significant number of people suffering attribute their pain to circumstances, events, and seemingly random misfortunes. However, I began to sense that the Iyengar method itself was the true source of their agony.

This realization fascinated me. Iyengar, after all, had gained international acclaim for his therapeutic successes and was renowned as a master pain-reliever. But this reputation was rooted in India.

Outside India, I struggled to reconcile such achievement and fame with the reality I observed.

I realized that Iyengar was a genius—he was a brilliant craftsman, but not an industrialist. that is, he did not know how to reproduce results on a large scale. So, his work was not a method because it was not replicable. To be a method, what is created must be replicable.

The overarching feeling was that the work I was encountering was really rough work. There was something very different happening between what Iyengar delivered and what these people who orbited around him could deliver. So, I didn't transfer the responsibility of what I was encountering to Iyengar himself. It was more that the practitioners surrounding him lacked the depth and precision of his work, which further reinforced my view that this was not a true method.

In Italy, amidst so many individuals in evident pain, I began to discern a deeper incoherence. It became clear that the practitioners of Iyengar Yoga, were immersed in a universe replete with rules, yet seemed disconnected from a long-term vision of well-being.

When I talked to Theresa about this, she confirmed that many were indeed grappling with pain. Yet there was a pervasive reluctance to address this issue openly, likely due to the almost devotional reverence surrounding Iyengar. That made my hair stand on end.

And then, I myself was adjusted by Gabriela when in a forward folding position. It resulted in one of the most severe injuries of my life, a ligament rupture in the back of my thigh that would take years of effort to heal. I realized then that many experienced practitioners lacked the sensitivity to accurately read bodies. Although Gabriela was the event's promoter, it was clear to me that she lacked attunement not only with me, but also with Theresa and others.

This adjustment severely restricted me and upon returning to Brazil, I had to be taken off the plane in a wheelchair...

By this time, during the meeting in Italy, I had already changed my plans. I had previously decided to go to the United States the following year, 1999, accepting Theresa's invitation. However, after the incident and injury, I reconsidered. With a renewed focus on the issue of pain, I decided to travel abroad for in-depth research, not limited to yoga. This time, my destination would be England.

Embarking on six months of intensive study, Francisco set up his base in Exeter, located 176 miles (282 km) south of London. The city, renowned for its medieval Gothic Anglican cathedral, was also home to Masterworks International, a prominent school of polarity therapy. This institution was founded by Phil Young and Morag Campbell, who are considered intellectual heirs to the pioneering work of Randolph Stone.

I went there to study natural health from another perspective, precisely because I no longer saw the point in continuing to look for what I was not finding in yoga. I had already discovered in Brazil, in a semi-empirical way, Randolph Stone's works. His research work began in the 1920s and 30s and reached its final form in the 1950s. There are two very striking things in his work.

First, he compiled key concepts from all major traditions, which he referred to as energy or electromagnetic medicine. He drew from ancient Greco-Roman traditions as well as more fundamentalist Chinese and Indian practices. He translated concepts from these traditions into a Western framework, and then combined ideas from osteopathy, chiropractic, and naturopathy, creating a cohesive and efficient system. He introduced these groundbreaking ideas to the public in the 1950s, well ahead of other scientists who only began discussing similar concepts in the 1980s and 1990s. For instance, Jean-Pierre Barral, an osteopath, only started teaching his visceral manipulation technique in the United States in 1985.

I dove into a period of intensive learning. It was a private course. In the morning, I had theoretical classes with a teacher, and in the afternoon, I had practical classes with another teacher. At night, I cleaned up my notes and processed what I learned.

I had already studied all of Stone's work as a self-taught student and realized that there were many good things. But I had never studied with someone knowledgeable. Stone had interpreted the techniques by himself and created a version of them. I was able to check at the school whether this work was correct.

But because I was alone and had a lot of free time, despite the intense course, I also had time to enter into the yoga scene in England. The yoga world there was deeply shaped by direct Indian influence. I frequently traveled to London, as it was home to many prominent figures in international yoga. I wanted to observe their work firsthand and understand what they were doing.

So, I attended classes, watched classes, watched bodies, and watched things happen. I attended several different schools and different styles of practice. I observed what I already knew in my body: that yoga existed in this delicate space where there was great potential for healing but also great potential for injury.

It was also during this period that an English method of chiropractic powerfully caught my attention: The McTimoney method.

John McTimoney was an artist, engraver, and technical illustrator who reproduced military aircraft and metallurgical parts for the British Air Ministry during World War II. Prior to this period, while working on a farm, he had a fall that left him paralyzed in the arms and struggling to walk. The threat of a risky spine surgery loomed over him. Fortunately, he was saved by an English chiropractor who had been trained in the United States by David Daniel Palmer, the founder of chiropractic practice in North America. This experience inspired John to devote himself to what was then considered a new therapeutic art, still largely unrecognized by conventional medicine, and without specialized schools in the United Kingdom.

Fortunately for McTimoney, a few years after World War II, Mary Walker, an English chiropractor, who also trained at Palmer's school in the United States, decided to introduce the teaching of chiropractic in her hometown, Oxford, towards the end of her life. Although she lacked the resources to open a formal school, she began offering private lessons to interested candidates. According to legend, recognizing John's great potential, Mary provided him with free mentoring, as he could not afford the tuition.

Certified in 1951, John embarked on an extraordinary career dedicated to modernizing, renewing, and advancing chiropractic practice. He established his own school in 1972 and, in 1979, lent his name to an association founded to support the ongoing evolution of what became recognized as a new branch of chiropractic: the McTimoney Chiropractic method.

It caught my attention because this was the first chiropractic work I encountered that wasn't approached from an American perspective.

The American view is often very mechanistic and segmented. Typically, if the problem is in the foot, American chiropractors work on the foot. If the issue is with the neck, they treat the neck. The American school does not consider a significant biomechanical or systemic logic.

This is not because Americans do not know. They know. But they have a theory of how to build the chiropractor's business. They don't want the person's problem solved. They want there to be, in a way, a codependency over time. But this is not sustainable. In this case, there is an apparent ethical issue, a fragile line between ethics and practice. The person who is dependent will never engage in the therapeutic process itself.

It is possible for people to enter the therapeutic process when they understand the benefits; when they understand the comfort that comes after they enter firmly into the pain.

The work of McTimoney is systemic, much like Stone's work is systemic. I understood that things need a systemic approach to work. The energy medicine I encountered was also effective in altering physical structures.

My time in England was incredible. I really enjoyed the theory, the study, the observations, and the hands-on practice. When it ended, I returned to Brazil with increased confidence. I came back with the intention of opening new and larger classes because up to then I had only a single, experimental, small class. This was the class that I had used to develop a lot of these new things that I was doing.

About a year or so later, I accepted a new invitation from Theresa. The last time she had been to Brazil, which was before her trip to Italy, she had observed my experimental group. She had never seen a class like mine before. She said, "This thing you do is nothing I know. But it's terrific!"

She wanted me to work at her school. She tried to support me in getting a green card or an immigrant visa, and conquering America, and living a dream that she envisioned I might have: making it to America and living the Great American Dream.

But was that my intention?

No.

I accepted the invitation just because I wanted to see what was there and get to know a large, important American school like hers.

Theresa's really was such a school.

Francisco landed in New York with a sharper critical spirit than ever. His previous experiences in Italy and England had illuminated the gaps he observed in the conventional yoga practice commonly accepted within Western society. These experiences had in the very least, opened a small portal for him, hinting at ways to address these voids.

He also disembarked with his spirit open, ready to embrace the positive surprises that might come his way.

I ended up teaching a lot of very interesting people. I worked with an audience that was open to new ideas and challenged me intellectually. I interacted with Americans who had a progressive worldview, quite different from the stereotypical image of the average conservative, consumerist American.

Many professors and students from the famous Juilliard School of Performing Arts attended these classes, including musicians, actors, singers, and dancers. Also present were scientists, researchers, and technicians from Bell Labs in the Center for Industrial Research and Scientific Development, which is historically associated with the inventor of the telephone, Alexander Graham Bell. And professionals from the financial market and marketing sectors attended. This was an America far removed from the stereotypical images of many people.

And I also had a room to lose myself in—the yoga library of Theresa's school. It was an extraordinary library that I had never imagined could exist.

I also had the space to teach. I assisted several teachers with their classes, taught my own classes, and provided private lessons because the school offered this service. My classrooms quickly began to fill up. This was largely because I had the freedom to do what I wanted, just as I had been doing in Brazil. I introduced the experimentation that had been happening in Curitiba into Theresa's school.

What guided the experimentation had a common inquisitive destiny. There were several people involved, each carrying their own specific issues. But what was the common denominator among them? What does everyone need, universally?

My limited command of English at the time posed a significant challenge. The difficulty in verbal expression forced me to develop strong non-verbal communication and body reading skills, both in groups and individually. This refined my perception of the classroom environment and gave me the ability to quickly read the dynamics of the room.

This quality of observation is truly fascinating. It allows you to determine whether individuals are genuinely ready to pursue their own liberation or if they are caught in an addictive cycle, avoiding pain rather than confronting it.

There is this powerful trend today. It already existed at that time. The doctor wants you to be pain-free. You don't want pain either. However, the more doctors try to deliver an analgesic to you, and the more you take it, the closer to an inevitable and debilitating pain you will be. The idea of not feeling is, in essence, what furthers sickness.

When the mind turns to "I don't want Ed to feel," it handcuffs Ed to the chain of body deterioration. The only possible rescue is movement. This movement needs to be built in a certain way so that Nature can reorganize itself. This usually involves diving into pain.

Of course, the dive must be done like a spaceship re-entering Earth's orbit. Success depends on the right speed, angle, timing, and numerous other carefully calculated factors. But the only way to return to Earth—to better health and wellness—is a path through pain, not around it.

As my understanding of my work deepened during my time in New York, I continued to grapple with significant pain. The incident in Italy haunted me for years but ultimately continued to shape my perspective on yoga and its methodologies.

When I arrived In New York, I brought with me insights from observing so-called yoga methods in London. I recognized that each approach had gaps, primarily due to a lack of understanding of biological identity. Every practitioner was forced into the same mold, repeating standard patterns. While these patterns were useful for some, many of whom became prominent yoga teachers, their success was often due to their physical performance rather than true understanding.

I was shocked to learn that many renowned teachers experienced episodes of anger, domestic violence, and depression. I also suspected that certain yoga methods could lead to hip issues, a concern that was confirmed years later when some teachers required hip prostheses.

It was absurd that many of these people were justifying their poor health outcomes from yoga as a genetic issue. Epigenetics scholars had already highlighted that genes are not definitive determinants. They *represent possibilities, which can be influenced by lifestyle, mental and emotional attitudes, and environmental factors. The world was beginning to acknowledge this new understanding, yet yoga, instead of being a cutting-edge health practice, was increasingly seen by me as fanciful and outdated. It lacked updates in technical knowledge and failed to provide health benefits, except in a few niche areas.*

In my eyes, this approach represented a form of brutality, lack of self-respect, intelligence, critical thought, and vision of the process. That's why by the time I reached New York I had lost respect for the prevailing mentality within the yoga community, with the exception of a few niche areas.

I arrived certain that I would witness a display of ignorance, and that's precisely what I saw. From the start, I understood that American yoga is an interpretation of yoga by a consumerist and anxious society. Yoga has become an industry, focused on selling mats, clothes, and accessories. While it's acceptable for yoga to be an industry, the problem lies in its lack of foundational understanding.

I didn't see American yoga as a place that takes care of each individual student. I saw yoga destroying bodies and overloading the nervous system. It was easy to understand, from a natural point of view, why many practitioners and teachers alike were depressed.

People were there because they applied American ideals to yoga: competitiveness, discipline, and overcoming. They imposed these ideals on the mechanical complexity of yoga positions without considering the individual's life history, biological individuality, or traumatic experiences. This approach created a time bomb, resulting in thousands of injuries. They gave rise to an absurd maxim: that acquiring injuries after long-term yoga practice was inevitable and could be attributed to one's karma.

Karma has become justification for the incompetence of teachers and practitioners. I had already noticed signs of this in Europe because there were many Americans doing yoga there. I had already seen this population super hurt and injured. When I noticed this, I immediately thought, "Ok, I'm going to the United States to see a mess and amazing bodies. But I won't see yoga, balance, peace of mind, healthy bodies that support mental maturation, and incredible aging. I'm going to see anxiety, pure anxiety."

I don't know if the Indians fueled the American market with what Americans crave—effort—because effort sells better, or if the Americans distorted what they received from India. My feeling is that they simply delivered what sold well: spiritual opium in the form of physical exertion. True balance, nervous system regulation, calmness, and maturity were not widely appealing or effective in spreading yoga.

I observed behaviors in some teachers that greatly displeased me. I met individuals who had been teaching yoga for 30 years and traveled to India every year to spend three months there. I couldn't help but think, if these instructors are away for three months each year, what happens to their students? There seemed to be a lack of responsibility and quality control in the delivery of their teaching. These teachers didn't hold regular classes or have a consistent student base. Instead, they primarily made money by promoting workshops.

And wow—I attended some of these workshops. At one of them, I discovered that the teacher had never met any of the participants before. As a result, he just vomited content no one was prepared to receive in their physical structure.

I had a student slightly older than me who came to take classes with me at Theresa's but didn't enjoy it. We didn't see eye to eye. Sometime later, he told me he had an accident during a workshop. Although he was quite flexible, he fell from an extreme position and broke his shoulder. He needed to undergo several surgeries to reconstruct the ligaments. This happened because the instructor did not understand the proper process or adhere to standards of sustainability.

I immediately understood something very important for my entire life. I understood that delivery has to happen every day in the classroom. I began to associate my clinical practice with the classroom.

Brazil is a seductive country, so it made sense that Theresa asked me to help her set up workshops here because she wanted to start doing things in Brazil. However, I replied,

"Definitely not!"

Because the workshop culture is one of the main cancers in the American market.

Theresa had a feeling that a lot of things were wrong. She had a lot of chronic pain. She also understood that there was an emotional and mental dysregulation. I understood that this all had to do with yoga, but she had built her life on yoga as she knew it, you know?

She was super-receptive to my observations. But I still approached her carefully on this. I was still forming my understanding of it all, also. I told her,

"For certain yoga positions to be effective and not cause future pain, even for people who seem to have natural flexibility, they need to be developed through a healing, therapeutic approach. This approach focuses on expanding healthy energy potential. Unfortunately, this is not always the case. Externally, your posture may appear perfect, but your eyes reveal the pain you are in. Internally, your organs may be struggling, leading to various health issues. These health problems can be directly linked to your practice."

To my surprise, she gave me an incredible answer,

"I think so too, but I'm too afraid to admit it to myself."

That's when I realized there was an elephant in the room that no one was addressing. In yoga, proper posture is crucial. It can help you age gracefully without pain or disability. However, people need to learn how to build this path correctly. They often think that posture is just about the shape or the appearance. In reality, posture is about function, biomechanical organization, and the optimization of human potential.

Theresa was the first person to understand that. As a result, there was some relief and an improvement in her condition. This was the initial recognition that other Americans would later share. It was they, the Americans, who would teach me that there was special value in what I was doing,

"You have hands that truly understand. Your touch, whether in the classroom or elsewhere, carries information, therapeutic content, and healing results."

It was time for Francisco to return home. To fulfill his desire to expand his classes of students. It was time for him to realize he was in the midst of a creative journey. He was preparing to offer his unique and exclusive contribution to the world of health: Kaiut Yoga.

It is also time for this narrative to shift in time and place, pausing the history of the method for a moment to explore the evolving story of Francisco's life. A story that runs parallel to that of Kaiut Yoga, yet is deeply intertwined like Siamese twins, forever connected.

You see, Francisco may appear to be two different people, the one immersed in yoga and the one outside of it. This is a trick played by our minds, of course. In reality, he is a single, complex human being, just like you and me. To truly understand how Kaiut Yoga came to be—and Francisco—I invite you to take a step forward in this narrative adventure and dive into waters where these intersecting storylines come together.

7

The Paradise—and Purgatory—
of the 4th and 7th Houses

We can draw an analogy between the concept of "houses" in astrology and the idea of parallel plots in films to frame the themes of this coming chapter of Francisco's story.

In an astrological chart, houses correspond to major areas of life a person's life or domains of human experience, such as career, family, or health. The twelve houses are always active and operate in parallel with one another, although the influence and prominence of a house in a person's life at a given time varies depending on a number of factors. Similarly, in good movies, while there is a primary linear narrative tied to a central event, there are also subplots that weave through parallel timelines, actions, and places.

To grasp the profound and often complex nature of human experience you must engage your thoughts and emotions in a spiral-like motion rather than linear one. In this state, past, present, and future intertwine, creating a dynamic interplay across multiple planes of time and place. It's in this dance that clarity emerges—a light breaks through, illuminating the vibrant pulse of life and shattering the rigid, polarized perspectives that often limit our understanding of existence.

Real life is multifaceted, composed of many themes, yet one appears to be universal across all lives, as echoed in astrology and good storytelling: the history of relationships. This theme is so central in astrology that it is addressed by more than one house. The 4th house pertains to the family, home, and one's roots, while the 7th house focuses on intimate partnerships. Through such intimate relationships—with parents, romantic partners, or children—we have the opportunity to discover and build a vital side of who we are. In this house, both joy and pain await us.

Antonio:

Francisco was 15 years old. My wife went to talk to the girl's mother. And warned her,

"My son has been coming to your house to see your daughter. Don't let it happen. This can be a problem."

After a while, the girl appeared pregnant. The parents knocked at my door. I was firm, "Look, here's the thing. My wife went to your house, warned your wife: 'don't let my son into the house.' But she did let him in, didn't she?"

Her husband was there, quiet.

I went on,

"That's the result. But that's okay. Let her have her pregnancy. We will do everything to help her and the child. You will have our full support, everything that is necessary within our reach. Now, there won't be a wedding. No! No one is getting married here!"

It would have been a tragedy for everybody. It was going to be very heavy for Francisco, as it was. But it wasn't his fault.

We had no way of knowing at the time, but it soon became clear to all of us that his focus is yoga. He got into it of his own free will, went through many obstacles, a lot of difficulty, but he never gave up. So, we also took up this focus, trying to help in whatever way we could to continue along that path, to this day. [Getting married and starting a family at that time] …could have been a disaster!

There would come a time, however, when Francisco would welcome starting a family.

I didn't envision a traditional family at the start of my adult life, unlike many men who dream of having children. My north has always been yoga. I had a very crazy connection with work, with the volume of work and with professional desires much more than anything else.

But Maria Alice and I were teenage sweethearts. However, we lost touch at some point, because she lived in the countryside, and I lived in Curitiba.

After a few years of being really involved with yoga, we reconnected kind of by chance. Then there was a fire of passion... We ended up dating more seriously, then we moved in together. And then, when I was twenty-six years old, Ravi happened.

That was a moment of surprise because he was not a planned child. But when it happened, it was super welcome. In a way, both she and I knew he was coming... then, there he was... the pregnancy was very nice, very well enjoyed, you know?

What I most admired about Maria Alice was her strong professional orientation. She worked in education and for me this is very important. The easiest thing for me to admire in any person is their nature and their professionalism and dedication to work. However, when she became a mother, she disconnected from everything professionally. She became a full-time mother.

She was a fantastic mother of a small child, absolutely dedicated, available, a very good person, really. But the abandonment of her professional aspirations was a bucket of cold water for me. We gradually disconnected, until we separated, when Ravi was three to four years old.

We had normal shared custody, so there was no problem. I stayed with Ravi two nights a week. We alternated weekends with him. This parenting thing was very pleasant for me. Taking him to school, picking him up from school, keeping up with homework, bathing, brushing his hair... I think it's in coexistence that you strengthen ties and educate.

When he turned seven, he came to live with me full-time. I was already dating Luciana and then we set up a structure for him. A room, toys. When Luciana got pregnant with Malu, the idea of him having a sister was positive and very impactful. Even at that time Ravi began to demonstrate that he has this very strong orientation to family ties and building a family.

Shortly after my separation from his mother, Ravi took a fall on the school playground. Then, a phase of great pain began. It was pain, pain, pain. We took him to a pediatrician and orthopedic specialist. We eventually found out that he has a degenerative genetic disease, Legg-Calvé-Perthes Disease.

We knew that Maria Alice had something of the same nature. It was very common in the interior for this disease to happen. If it wasn't severe, the families didn't even find out, the child dealt with the pain alone. Ravi´s mother had this memory of having taken a fall in childhood and then she had a big difference between her right and left leg. There was a big difference in her hips too.

But Ravi's case was very severe. I started researching, understanding that this is a very difficult disease and that it impacts many people. In the initial phase, there is only one thing to do: rest.

Even so, I fought the idea that nothing I could do would be useful. I started to apply manual work to the soft tissue that I had learned in my training in natural health. Every night I put him to sleep doing something therapeutic, trying to relax and discharge his nervous system.

When the initial shock phase of the disease subsided, which typically happens around the age of eight or nine, I began a rehabilitation program with him. By that time, Ravi had already spent numerous years without a functioning body. Attending school proved to be extremely difficult. But since he couldn't do anything physically, he developed a very focused and very rigid personality. If he went to a party with friends and couldn't get on the trampoline, he would simply suppress his desire to join in. Despite his limitations, he retained a positive manner, working to cultivate a resilient personality.

I started a program so that he could develop an enchantment for the use of the body. I brought teachers from various sport disciplines to our home. And when my trips to the United States began, and he was a teenager, I started taking him along, so he could experience this universe of yoga more closely.

During our time in the U.S., he proved to be very charismatic and made friends easily. I believe that the culture of freedom, nature, sports, and outdoor life he encountered there was very important for *him. For instance, he really enjoyed learning to ski and picked it up very quickly, which shows how impactful the experience was for him.*

He developed an engaging and inclusive personality. Rather than going out, he preferred inviting friends over. He enjoyed hosting Sunday lunches and sleepovers at home. The nightlife did not appeal to him. His circle of friends, which started in childhood and expanded through school and Colorado, was always growing and inclusive, never excluding anyone.

I developed several therapeutic techniques for him. I created resources to minimize the impact that the disease could have on his adult life. And this was a great success, because this is a disease that in fact generates a pathological rigidity in adults, a rigidity that Ravi fortunately never developed.

Legg-Calvé-Perthes is a disease where there is insufficient blood supply to the upper part of the femoral growth plate, near the hip joint. The ultimate origin of this deficit of blood supply is still a mystery. The child may suffer serious hip damage that eventually results in permanent arthritis.

After a few years, Ravi had already overcome the most critical phase of the disease. Then, the tumultuous divorce I had with Luciana occurred, an absurd situation that also affected him, especially because he was very close to his sister, Malu.

I had briefly met Luciana, a while before we entered a relationship. She left Brazil to live abroad. After some time, when passing through here, she came to see me,

"Look, your work is incredible. I haven't seen anything like this, where I am living now. But I'm going to return to Brazil soon. We could open something together..."

In retrospect, I realize I was naïve. For the first time, I experienced someone genuinely appreciating my work and talent, and I got charmed by this. By this time, my work was already consistent and growing. I had already been through the New York period at Theresa's school and had traveled to Europe. I had about 80 or 100 students. We started dating, and then we moved in together. I was 30 years old.

I don't know if it was because of my separation from Ravi's mother. But I felt there was a different movement inside of me. I wanted to be married and start a family—so I married Luciana.

It was not a good marriage. It was filled with conflicts. We never lived very well together. It was more of a working partnership. Luciana supported me a lot in technical and intellectual creation. My work grew significantly in Curitiba, and soon, the expansion to the United States also began. I started to travel a lot, twice a year. These trips involved long projects, and I was away for months. This was almost like a drug. It had a sedative effect because the attacks and conflicts ceased when I traveled. But when I returned home, I found myself missing being on the move. There was a sense of longing there, truly.

I could leave because she took care of some things at work. Shortly after my return, the conflicts would begin again. It was always like this, cyclical, you know?

I think my travels to the United States were the main factor that kept us together. They provided a distraction from the conflicts. When I returned, I missed home, but soon after, another conflict would arise, and shortly after that, I would travel again. It was a vicious cycle of avoiding the problem because the dynamics of life kept everyone distracted. This went on for years.

Another important factor was that the business side of my work had become vibrant and thriving. Despite this, Luciana was not very competent in management. She fought with the teachers, the accountant, and practically everyone involved. Because of this, I had to get involved in the financial aspects of the business, which is hugely unpleasant for me.

The business side has never been my calling, it's just not in my nature. I never had the nature to make money. I have no conflict with that. It's okay if it's like that for you, I don't see a problem with that. But for me it's a crass desire, it doesn't fulfill me. It's a desire that takes me away from what organizes me and what I'm passionate about. And it's a lot of work!

I like creating. What enchants me is the result, it's the human interaction, it's the classroom, the production of content and knowledge. I don't take any hours out of the classroom, or from my study and practice time, for anything. If you invite me to a meeting or to a type of conversation that will prevent me from doing what I want to do well, I don't have time for you.

Along with this distraction from traveling, which deprived me of seeing how unhealthy that relationship was, there was a huge volume of work. I had a hard time regulating this. I took on an absurd volume of commitments, one after the other. As I love what I do, I don't see the weekend as most people do. The weekends are an opportunity to prepare content, record a class, organize another event.

My work is my passion, and my passion was my madness. I never reached Friday nights feeling tired and wondering: "Oh, my God, what am I going to do this weekend?" This is because of a choice I made long ago—rooted in my story of pain—to achieve a limitless body and a limitless mind. I love feeling that I am at the extreme of everything—performance, practice, study, and quality. Everything.

I thought weekends were boring. But this had a consequence on my family, many times, because I had no limits, but other people do. I didn't feel a lack of energy, but other people lack energy.

Luciana was not competent in the classroom either. She had no personal connection to yoga, yet she began to teach. However, she was very charismatic and knew how to communicate effectively with people. This side of her made a significant difference but also created the illusion that she was a good teacher.

This led to big quarrels between us. I said,

"What do you mean? You are teaching yoga? But you don't even get close to a mat! You don't practice; you don't study..."

It was ridiculous. I had witnessed similar behavior in past relationships, but it wasn't until Luciana that I truly grasped the significance. Whenever something like this occurred, it was a clear indication that I should walk away. Women I had been in previous relationships with, treated dating me as a way to enhance their image or skills... as if it improved their resumé as a teacher or yogini... "I date this guy, and he's great, so I also reap the benefits."

I gave Luciana space because our relationship was very complicated for me to assert myself in. It was a big mistake because she assumed authority she did not possess. She was like a clone, walking behind me in the shadows, using it to her advantage.

If the outlook of this relationship gradually became gloomy, it would darken even further. In a way that Francisco could never have imagined.

I really wanted to be a father once more. I really wanted to have a daughter this time. Luciana didn't want to have children. But she got pregnant. It was a shock for her when Malu was born. And it was surprising for me to find out that Luciana was a non-maternal person, she had no maternal instinct. It surprised me because my previous reference was Maria Alice, who was such a maternal person.

That caught my attention, but I didn't give it much weight because it was convenient for me. I had always been a very maternal father to Ravi, so Malu's arrival provided me with a space that I welcomed. A space to experience again the joys of giving the baby their first bath, of being present during the early years, of living through those precious moments.

When Ravi moved in with us, I took the two of them, him and Malu, to school and brought them home from school. I had a super organized routine, and as I was not teaching at night, I was able to make them both dinner, bathe them, brush their hair, and put them to bed. Only after that, at the end of my day, would I practice my yoga.

As time went by, a year before the divorce, I realized that our marriage had become a very sick relationship. Fights escalated, growing increasingly hostile. When I returned from trips to the United States, none of the agreements we had established had been honored. I wanted to spend time with the children, but I would come home to find that Luciana had taken them on trips for days on end. Financial issues also began to escalate, creating further confusion. She even started cutting off the flow of money from the business to me.

One night I was sitting at the table, sipping my glass of wine. She arrived on the other side, started saying some things and opened an argument. I held the glass in my hand, I thought, "my God, this again?"

I suddenly became quiet. You know when you are distracted from a situation, and you don't even know what the other person is talking about? She started screaming; really screaming. She started screaming and walking backward as if I was physically assaulting her. But I was just sitting there. I immediately realized that the environment was becoming completely unsafe. I thought to myself, "wow, this situation is escalating. She is going crazy for good. Soon she will throw herself on the ground, and I will be seen as the violent person, even though I was not involved."

That same night, or the next morning, I don't remember, I left. I checked in at a hotel. I understood that there was no longer a minimum condition for dialogue. I was living in a horror movie. However, there were positive aspects in this marriage. There was a daughter. In cases like this, you are reluctant to embrace the idea that the person is unbalanced to this degree.

As soon as Malu was born, I had had one of the most creative phases of my life. My method was already under development. So, at this stage, I designed many lesson plans, sequences for applying techniques, new accessories. I dreamed a lot, very often I woke up with new ideas. I already used bolsters in various ways, for example, but one night I dreamed of my hands clasped under a bolster.

While bolsters are a standard yoga accessory, used by teachers of different styles, the intertwining of the fingers under the bolster when the practitioner is lying down, is specifically associated with the logic of the Kaiut Yoga method.

Sometimes, I woke up at dawn because Malu was a baby who stayed awake many nights. I took the time to test something I had just invented, trying some new idea. Another emotional memory linked to Malu is that she was born prematurely, 15 days after my mother's death. It was a very intense period of strong and disparate emotions. When she was born, Ravi asked to come and live with us too, which was the beginning of very close relationship between him and Malu. It was very difficult for Luciana to be a mother, but I was familiar with the exercise of fatherhood and motherhood. This made me change my daily routine, creating a very good family dynamic with the children.

Later I would discover that Luciana's absurd scene that night was a classic act of "parental alienation." A lawyer of mine explained to me the kinds of things that can happen, for example, the woman makes an appointment at a mall with her husband, whom she is separating from. She turns on her cell phone, throws herself on the ground, and films herself getting up, screaming that it was the man who assaulted her. It happens every day, a thousand times a year, in Brazil.

The reality is the alienation had begun well before that night, through her creating separation. I would go to pick up the children, and they would not be there. I'd be perplexed, unable to believe this could happen. I admired Luciana for certain attitudes and types of companionship at work. But suddenly, I found myself facing behavior that was not only ethically questionable but childish. The intelligence I once saw in her was no longer there. I didn't know who I was dealing with anymore. Hundreds of attempts at dialogue had come to nothing.

A long time before we reached a mutual agreement for divorce, she had an abdominal crisis and had to be rushed to the hospital. The doctor administered a cocktail of antibiotics, which was a shock to her system, and triggered a bipolar crisis.

From then on, bipolar crises made living together unbearable. Once, I took her to the United States. Traveling business class on an American Airlines flight, she drank and started talking harshly to a flight attendant. I thought this is going to suck. This woman is going to get thrown in jail when she lands in the United States. It took me a long time to calm her down.

Luciana started to defame me by telling Lúcia Torres, my first teacher at my yoga studio in Curitiba, and then several students, that I had another house with a mistress. This was absolutely crazy, as she was a woman who had never been betrayed.

We had many senior students at school. So, she victimized herself to them, cried, and said that I had had many lovers throughout the marriage. She co-opted these people. Thus, it killed a large part of the school's student base. And when I traveled, everything went absolutely crazy. Over time, the school would go bankrupt, and debts soared.

I started losing people who were passionate about the work and dozens of students who were deeply connected to the developing method. These students were passionate about the results they were achieving, not necessarily about the teacher. While it's obvious that there is a strong connection and empathy between the student and the teacher, the teacher should serve as a channel—a bridge that directly connects the student to the practice. This approach allows you to work with hundreds, even thousands of students, without being emotionally burned out. When students become passionate about the teacher, it creates a significant energetic weight, which is much less healthy for everyone involved. However, when the teacher acts as the bridge, it enables students to build a connection with the practice and the results they achieve.

My students had a very strong connection with me because of the work, the results, the healing, and the significant changes they experienced. However, many of these students were eventually alienated and distanced themselves after being targeted in deeply personal and sensitive ways. Luciana had a precise and calculated approach to these attacks. For example, if there was a 70-year-old student who was a very conservative Catholic, with deeply ingrained classical values, she would deliberately exploit this, planting doubts or framing events in a way that irreparably tarnished their perception of me.

I was somewhat myopic about all this for a long time, as I was deeply immersed in the development of the method. I didn't notice Luciana's backbiting and her targeting students she felt were vulnerable to her Machiavellian attacks. If I established a different relationship with someone, she would find a way to make contact with that person and tarnish my image.

When we had already decided to divorce, one day she had a breakdown and wanted to take Ravi away with her. His response was very firm. At 17 years old, Ravi was no longer a child but a young man with a solid personality. "Hey, wait a minute!" he said, putting up a clear boundary. Luciana practically kidnapped Malu. She fled Curitiba, leaving the yoga school in a significant amount of debt. That's when I began to truly understand what parental alienation is.

In legal terms, parental alienation refers to the harmful interference by a parent, grandparent, or other adult in a child or adolescent's psychological development, with the intent of damaging the relationship between the child and the other parent. While the definition is precise, clear, and objective, it fails to capture the full depth of the lived experience. You can only grasp the human dimension when fate thrusts you into it.

Alienating behavior begins when the couple is still together. I only understood this later when I started studying this subject. I consulted a lot of people, including lawyers, psychologists, and experts. I spent a lot of money on lawyers when Luciana's behavior escalated into the form of emotional and psychological violence against Malu.

In alienation, the child is deprived of what she has, of what she knows, of what she could have. She is gradually stripped of her good memories. She starts to see the episodes she experienced with love in a different way.

The alienator begins to build a manipulative discourse when they are still married, changing the child's perspective. Luciana managed to foster a hatred in Malu towards me. I noticed that Malu's reactions to me changed. It got to a point where she was no longer the child I knew before. I tried to dialogue with the child I had raised, but the response was no longer the same.

There was a period when I managed to see Malu regularly, in therapy. That came about through the force of justice and having my case examined by a very experienced expert. It was also super exciting for Ravi to see his sister again. The dynamic seemed to be working. But then Luciana found a way to get Malu out of there. And she disappeared for good.

I didn't see Malu for a long time. Then I found out her whereabouts—Luciana had fled to São Paulo with her. So, I opened an alienation process. At first, justice was favorable to me in the sense of determining the visitation process. But Luciana didn't fulfill it.

For more than a year I would pick up the car early in the morning in Curitiba, on the agreed day, and drive to São Paulo to see Malu. But then, when I would arrive at the scheduled time and place, no one would be there. Luciana hadn't taken her. In those situations, there's nothing to do... you have no one to turn to. What you can do is open a new lawsuit. A lawyer that has to set things in motion. But then more time goes by... more time not seeing Malu.

When you go to court in Brazil, in cases of alienation, you are faced with the slowness of justice. Every day of delay works in favor of the alienator and against the child.

When I first managed to take Malu to the experienced expert I mentioned earlier, the report was done very well, confirming the alienation. However, when the court process lacks the necessary speed, the alienator begins to gain the upper hand. Every extra hour and every extra day in not allowing the accused to visit the child works in favor of the alienator, providing additional opportunities to manipulate and influence the child's mind.

In Curitiba at that time, very little was known about parental alienation. The crime is multifaceted, with very complex legislation. Legally, the child is not supposed to lose contact with the accused parent. However, the child can be brainwashed, becoming more withdrawn each day. The longer the time away from the accused parent, the more the child's perspective is manipulated to align with that of the alienator.

In Brazil, almost ninety percent of the cases that relate to the Maria da Penha Law are not related to violence against women but to parental alienation and attempts to harm men. Leading experts in this field are aware of this phenomenon; it is statistically evident. The Maria da Penha Law is a fantastic and critical piece of legislation for a country where the justice system is often seen as unfair and incompetent. However, sadly it is being misused against its intended purpose.

Brazil is not like some other countries where a divorce cannot be finalized until child custody is agreed upon. In those countries, the child's welfare comes before anything else. Here, it's a battle, and as time passes, the child suffers more damage, becoming increasingly trapped in a place of suffering with no way out. The child is not just deprived of a father or mother, but of all the people she loves, and those people are deprived of her. The systemic violence is immense. In the long term, it is known that such children tend to suffer from depression, and suicide rates are very high.

I fought hard and spent a lot of money on lawyers, experts, and specialists—with no results. Except for the first action, which involved an expert who confirmed the case as one of parental alienation. This expert recommended, as she did to all parents and legal professionals, that I watch the documentary A Morte Inventada [The Invented Death]. *It portrays an intense and manipulative process, exactly like what Malu had been experiencing.*

Directed by Alan Minas, the Brazilian documentary details seven dramatic cases, including stories of false accusations, the ineffectiveness of the justice system, and a father who, despite having official authorization for custody, had to orchestrate police action worthy of a Hollywood movie to retrieve his children. One of the most emotionally impactful stories is that of a girl who spent 11 years living without her father, caught in the cruel trap set by the alienator. This is a classic situation where the child forms a pact of loyalty with the guardian, driven by emotional and material dependence.

Produced in 2009, the documentary has been shown at numerous national events promoted by the justice sector. It is also available for free on various YouTube channels, with more information on the production company's website, Caraminhola Filmes.

In São Paulo, Luciana filed a complaint against me under the Maria da Penha Law, alleging that I was hanging around her house and making her feel threatened. However, on the date she mentioned, I was actually in Curitiba, in a classroom with 60 students, trying to repair the damage she left behind.

I don't know if it was her intention or not but invoking the Maria da Penha Law postponed all legal processes and became a significant tool of alienation throughout Malu's life. I had a witness who could confirm I was in Curitiba, but the judge did not accept their testimony. It was shocking to experience such a terrible interaction with the justice system, which should, above all, protect the child.

When I found out which school Malu was attending in São Paulo, I went there to try to see her, following the advice of the alienation expert and my lawyer. They suggested I speak with the school administration, as some schools are more pro-family and don't simply believe everything the alienators say. When I arrived at the school, and Luciana found out I was there, she hurriedly grabbed Malu, causing a scene by claiming I was going to be violent with our daughter. She fled through the back, taking Malu with her. This put the school administration in a difficult position, as no one is prepared to handle such situations.

The years passed and then...

I was in São Paulo, in Vila Madalena, the city's charming neighborhood known for its bars, restaurants, and bohemian lifestyle.

I was there with a lawyer I was dating at the time. We were shopping when a sudden storm erupted.

It was lunchtime, and we entered a restaurant to shield ourselves from the rain and enjoy a meal. We went in laughing at the situation, having had a very fun morning. The restaurant was crowded. Many people were standing, but we managed to get a table.

As the maître d' brought the wine I ordered, I suddenly saw Malu standing, passing behind him. She looked at him and then her gaze met mine...

She was super spontaneous and came toward me. I stood up.

"Hi, dad!"

"Hi, daughter!"

At this moment, we connected with very genuine emotion. The emotion that came from her crossed the barrier of everything we had experienced.

I hadn't noticed that Luciana was also in the restaurant. She came running up behind me, grabbed Malu violently by the arm, and pointed her finger at me. She threatened me, screaming that I had a Maria da Penha order against me, that I was dangerous, and that I couldn't get close to Malu.

Luciana dragged Malu to the door, the rain pouring down outside. Malu was paralyzed, in shock, staring at the rain as if she were catatonic. My girlfriend at the time, who was not only a lawyer but mother also, and who had nothing to do with this story, looked on perplexed at the absurd scene unfolding before her.

That was the last time I saw Malu.

8

There's Always Another Day

There is always—or almost always—a day after, in life. All, or almost all the dramas of our destiny, when we are pressured from all sides, present us with the choice to shake off the dust and move forward, or sink into the mud of problems that lead nowhere. Extreme tests, especially when they affect multiple houses of our existence, can cause us to die inside, compromising our journey of growth as human beings. Alternatively, extreme tests can serve as leverage to elevate us to a higher realm of possibilities. As a popular Brazilian saying goes, these are moments "when the jaguar goes to the pond to drink water"; in Brazilian Portuguese, "a hora da onça beber água." It is a time of vulnerability when one must confront challenges directly if they arise; there is no escape.

Both joy and dejection are available options just beyond the path of pain. The choice is always ours.

There was a final hearing at the very beginning of the COVID-19 pandemic, in 2020, to which Malu was invited by the judge. My lawyers advised me not to attend, as they suspected that even the judge would be shocked by the absurdity of the situation. And they were right! It is absolutely absurd! However, I had already decided not to go because I had reached my limit with it all. I didn't want to risk transferring any sense of hurt to the victim. Because Malu is a victim.

As I had already tried everything possible to reverse what was happening, I had gone beyond my limits. When the hearing occurred, I decided to accept life as it was presenting itself. I chose to be available if Malu sought me out. I decided that this whole crazy episode would not make me ill. I wouldn't let it tarnish my health or live in anger or hurt. This situation would not define me as a person.

I kept some important records of this story, though not with me. I entrusted them to the office I hired to handle it. I decided that I would be happy. I chose to accept everything that needed to be accepted, everything I couldn't change, including my mistakes. I resolved to use this episode to become a more mature, better, and more capable person. I chose to plunge into the eye of the pain. The pain of missing Malu is something I have to welcome every day. However, pain and suffering does not mean you can no longer experience fantastic moments in life or build a career or rescue your health.

The degree of despair, torment, effort, and energy expenditure I endured, including the dozens and dozens of trips I made to São Paulo—all of it was very taxing. On the day of the hearing, I had tremendous tachycardia; but I decided it wouldn't ruin my health.

The evil done against Malu is immense, but if I let anger take over, what will I be angry at? A person? I could choose to see it as Luciana's actions, but I don't think any personal malice can match the scale of what happened. Behind this evil is something much bigger—she has a disease.

What am I going to be angry about? The disease? Letting anger consume me is illogical. There's no way I can be angry about a disease.

When looking back at all this, I recognize I didn't have the maturity I have now. I remember one day, for the first time, opening up to someone at the yoga school in Curitiba. I had kept quiet with the students, not revealing anything about my torment. I decided however to talk with my friend and first teacher at the school, Lúcia Torres. I told her everything behind Luciana's scandals.

"And what are you going to do, Francisco?"

"There's nothing to do, Lúcia. I have consulted all the experts I could. Luciana's attack is heavy. There is no loophole to open a defamation or slander lawsuit. There is nowhere to catch her. So, I decided to sit down and work—work, work!"

I started to work more than ever: to rescue the school, get new students, and train teachers, while also keeping the activities in the United States going. I worked amidst all the chaos—Luciana's attacks, judicial notifications, the execution of actions, the search for Malu, and all the consultations with specialist professionals.

I turned to my practice. The school was already being recommended by many doctors, and I was working with very complex situations, managing risks with significant results. Many orthopedists, neurologists, and angiologists recognized the school—referred to as the Yoga of Praça da Espanha ["The Spanish Square"] in the Batel neighborhood—as something unique and iconic with safe results.

Teaching offered me the only moments of peace I had. It allowed me to focus on others and get out of my issues for a while. This focus on others during each class gave me a great sense of organization and relief.

I decided not to give myself a single minute with an empty head when I wasn't teaching. I started reading one or two books a week, listening to audiobooks, and watching movies—anything to prevent myself from falling into a place of pain, anguish, anger, or conflict.

Ravi, although still very young, began to help me with many practical things in everyday life. When things settled down in Curitiba and the school started to run smoothly, I focused more intensely on my international career. In addition to the United States, an opportunity arose in Toronto, Canada, followed by Amsterdam in Europe.

The method I had developed began to mature. In courses, I started to explain in technical detail what I had initially developed intuitively. I had to articulate logically what I was doing so that the method could be replicable. From then on, I reorganized myself as a person and teacher, along with the method. I created a substantial volume of technical and intellectual resources that elevated the method to a new level.

Then I realized that what had already been an incredible career with amazing results—and what was already a significant school and method—had become something far beyond my original expectations.

A spiritual inclination even started to emerge, rooted in very simple ideas of acceptance. Understand the pain, accept the pain. Recognize that being angry with someone with a psychiatric issue won't get you anywhere. Understand and accept that loss cannot define the rest of your life.

Putting all this into perspective and maturing internally was the unexpected silver lining of losing Malu.

The sacrifices we endure through loss and the trials of extreme tests can become a powerful force in deepening our awareness of who we are and what we are doing in this world. This process can often require us to open the floodgates of perception, wherein new visions of one's potential and life trajectory may arise. As a result, we may also see start perceiving and engaging with reality through lenses that are distinct from the vast majority of people. Arguably, this is where Francisco found himself.

This journey of understanding, as you already know, traverses planes of time and places that dance before us like a pendulum of discoveries, swinging back and forth. It is a spiral of continuous coming and going.

Ravi:

I always got along well with my father, but there was also a lot of conflict between us. As a child, my relationship with my mother was light. She was my safe haven, no matter what happened. If I needed her, she was always there. She was the lightest figure in my life. However, my relationship with my father and Luciana was difficult. They both had very strong opinions, and so did I, even from a young age. Additionally, Luciana had many clashes with my mother, which complicated things further.

I was a child and a teenager who had to deliver a lot. I had to get the best grades and do a thousand things. I always had a very good education, and my father allowed me a lot of freedom. However, it was an education with high demands and many rules. I had to achieve certain things to get what I wanted. For example, doing well in high school meant I could travel on vacation. Doing poorly meant staying home.

I learned to read and write in German at the Swiss-Brazilian School in Curitiba. I wasn't a very diligent student and often went to school reluctantly.

However, in the eighth grade, I achieved the best grades of my life, which allowed me to go on a graduation trip to the interior of Paraná. Thinking I could do anything since I had done well in school, I prepared for the trip with about six other classmates. We smuggled in some drinks.

We got caught and were expelled. I thought my father was going to kill me when he was called to the principal's office. But on the drive home, he turned to me and said,

"At least you had fun!"

The school, recognized and supported by both the Swiss government and the educational authority of the state of Paraná, has a faculty composed of Swiss and Brazilian teachers. The teaching is bilingual. This education must have been vital in shaping Ravi's cosmopolitan mind and openness to the world, even though he considers himself a less-than-diligent student.

I continued my studies at the Dom Bosco school, growing up with a lot of pain due to a degenerative disease known as Legg-Calvé-Perthes. The head of the femur on my right side is deformed. It doesn't fit into the acetabulum, where the femur articulates with the pelvis. Until I was 13, I limped. I couldn't run, jump, play, or do anything without pain, as all activity could worsen how the femur head would develop in the future.

My father insisted that I practice yoga repeatedly. Luciana also demanded a lot from me, in every aspect. As a child, I didn't understand. I saw their relationship was fraught with bad habits from the beginning. I viewed Luciana as a bad person and my father as an aggressive one. I witnessed many arguments and slamming of doors—it was constant aggression from one to the other. Luciana, however, took it to the next level with the situation with my sister, Malu. She lied, manipulated, and tried to create false narratives. My father didn't lie, but what led to my sister's extreme situation seemed to be planted by both of them. It's hard to convey this to my father directly.

I was mainly confused by what I saw as my father's extreme lack of control, which didn't match what I saw of him at the yoga school. There, he took great care in how he spoke with teachers and students, which contrasted sharply with his behavior during fights with Luciana.

I think my father wanted to be my teacher, but he couldn't accept it when I didn't do what he wanted. I perceived him as absurdly violent with me, emotionally. It took me years to understand that this absurdity had nothing to do with me. It had to do with his upbringing, his values, and the person he wanted me to become. It was about his emotional rigidity.

Because of his behavior, I remember once saying as a child,

"I hate yoga! I will never work with anything that has to do with you!"

I didn't like studying because sitting for long periods was unbearable; it hurt and made me anxious. At 13, when my hip joint condition solidified, I was able to come back to life. From then on, I started to love using my body.

At 15, I had my last pain crisis. I was with my girlfriend at the time and her mother at Prestinaria, a famous bakery in Curitiba. While sitting, the pain suddenly came on very strong. I went to the bathroom to stretch my leg, crying in pain, alone. I leaned against the bathroom wall, stretched both legs forward, and lowered my body, trying to relieve the pain behind my knee.

Nothing helped. I spent about 10 minutes there, crying. I had an inspiration and decided, internally, that I would never want to experience pain like that again. I remembered my father's words,

"You have to practice! You have to practice yoga!"

I practiced, but it often felt forced by him. Sometimes I rebelled,

"Damn, okay! You want me to do this, but I don't need it."

After that pain crisis however, my practice gained momentum. About two years later, I discovered bodybuilding. As a chubby teenager, I weighed 100 kilos

[220lbs]. I decided to compete, and by my first competition, I had dropped to 69 kilos [around 150lbs]. I became the champion of Paraná, then Brazilian champion. I competed in an amateur world championship in Hungary and placed tenth.

During my bodybuilding phase, I started working with my father. I chose to work with yoga, not to help him through his tumultuous divorce, but because of my condition. I saw people with the same problem I had who were disabled. Many were in wheelchairs, unable to walk, with hip prostheses and numerous surgeries. Yet, I was able to do what I wanted and was able to use my body to an incredible degree. Then I came across a report of a man on American TV who had the same disease as I did. He was in a wheelchair, discussing his life. It hit me hard. That could have been my life if I wasn't working on my body. I called my father,

"Dad, I understand what you do! It's so good! I want to work with you!"

The first thing I thought I wanted to do in life was to be a medical doctor. Having spent several periods in the United States with my father, I had applied for admission to schools there and had been accepted by some universities. He was thinking of emigrating permanently and was waiting for me there. I then called him again,

"Damn it, I hate blood. What am I going to do in the United States? Spend 12 years to study Medicine? I'm not going anymore. I'll see what I can do around here."

I enrolled in a business administration college at the age of 19. By the end of the first semester, I was starting to understand a bit of the subject. Then, one day, my father took me to an ATM in a shopping mall to withdraw money with my credit card and deposit it into the account of our company that managed the yoga school. I asked to see the numbers, and he showed them to me. I realized that we had been running a huge deficit for months. It was a financial mess. I told him,

"We're in deep trouble here! We need to organize this mess from now on!"

A while later, feeling unhappy in the business course, I went to spend a few days in the United States with a great friend of mine, Jackson, and his friend, Collins. We loved cooking together and often smoked marijuana while doing so, sharing our misfortunes. Then, out of the blue, Collins, stoned, suddenly said,

"Why don't you start studying cooking?"

We thought it was cool. We immediately started looking for schools around the world and found one we liked in New York, and another in Curitiba! I convinced Jackson, and he came here, spending two years with me. Together, we took the gastronomy course at the European Center, which partners with hotel and culinary schools in Switzerland.

Then I met Bruna. I got engaged and quit bodybuilding. I was happy with my life and had found the woman with whom I wanted to build a family. But I had to structure it properly.

Although I graduated in gastronomy, I never worked in the field. Instead, I began working intensely in yoga. I wanted to build a life with Bruna, make money, and pursue many ventures. I took care of managing my father's yoga business but soon became interested in teaching as well. I completed my father's teacher training program, and a year later, I started teaching.

Today, I am extremely grateful for my work as a teacher. I continue to manage my father's business, which remains my main job. Bruna and I now run the Kaiut Yoga school in the Batel neighborhood, the school that belonged to my father at Praça de Espanha. Bruna is also a teacher. She trained in other lines of yoga before joining us.

In 2017, when I started working with my father, we began to gradually develop a positive relationship. Our working relationship eventually grew into a strong personal bond.

The moment of truth. The key turning moment.

We are together today. We turned the key; changed the game for better. Partly because he changed, and partly because I took the step to change as well. He had to confront many of his inner demons, just as I had to deal with mine. Many years of therapy since I was young have helped me understand why family is so important to me and why forming a family the right way has always been my quest.

A therapeutic process with psychotherapist Antonio Carlos Jacobsen helped me a lot in understanding my father. It provided a clear panorama of his psyche. I learned that people do change but that the journey of maturation is tough without direction or therapy. My father, who achieved great success from a young age, saw his word as law.

My father was very strict, rigid with schedules, tasks, everything. I think this trait came from his father, my grandfather Antonio, who was a colonel in the Military Police. However, this same grandfather, with whom I work with closely every day, is now a light-hearted, calm man who talks about the joy of life. He is one of the healthiest people I know.

It's fantastic to see that my son, Bento, is developing a close relationship with his grandfather, similar to the one I have with mine. It's something I never imagined possible. My father and I never had that kind of bond. I feared he would disrespect my educational approaches for my son. But today, we are both much more open to dialogue, making everything flow smoothly. I am amazed at the person my father has become with my son.

My father's life was never easy at all. He was shot in the hip and lived most of his life in pain. He faced numerous setbacks. Nothing was ever simple for him. Yet, he always embodied yoga, and yoga always embodied him. Today, you can see how much this union benefits others. He is truly an admirable person, practicing yoga for six hours a day, constantly striving to develop and deliver more. This dedication makes him almost dysfunctional in everyday life outside of yoga. His level of commitment is extraordinary.

Why do I continue to dedicate myself to Kaiut Yoga?

Other than my physical situation, I witnessed my father's evolution through the practice. I saw the method transcend from merely a physical practice to something that profoundly impacted his mind. I observed him breaking old

FRANCISCO KAIUT with EDVALDO PEREIRA LIMA

behavior patterns, both in his work and in his relationships with us. He broke a long-standing family pattern of conflict that spanned multiple generations. It was a tough situation to be in, but I saw this transformation happen and realized—it was yoga.

The most enchanting aspect of the practice is my father's transformation. What he has created is a blessing, not just for our family but for many others. While mistakes can't be erased by a single success, they were necessary to achieve this profound accomplishment. The number of people we can help, lifting them from deep pain and suffering to give them a new life, is remarkable. We promote healthy aging and change lives. People who were on the brink of despair have found healing through this practice.

Life's processes are truly crazy.

"Crazy beautiful" seems fitting here, do you agree with me? This expression from Brazilian rock star Raul Seixas's song, "Maluco Beleza," perfectly encapsulates the unfolding of life's processes. There is a unique beauty that emerges when the dust of stormy paths settle, revealing the hidden light in the darkness and the sweet song that rises from the chaos.

In these moments, we realize that behind seemingly disruptive disorder lies the magic of a new order, weaving together meanings we couldn't have anticipated. On this map of life, we encounter individuals who cross our paths, initially seeming to play lasting roles. However, as the wheel of destiny turns, they guide us in directions we could never have imagined while still in the heat of the journey.

After a while, when everything was reorganized and the work in Curitiba boomed, also expanding abroad, my father decided to move to São Paulo, and not the United States.

There, he met Daniela, who turned out to be exactly what we needed at that moment. That's when his life really started to change. She was a blessing in his life, in mine, and in my grandfather's, because she brought a sense of calm. My father began to realize that many of his attitudes were ridiculous, and that's how others saw them too.

Daniela was always a wonderful person, a true gem. A yoga teacher herself, she embodied the most alternative, positive, and beautiful aspects of the yoga world. She was making my father a sweeter person.

They planned their wedding, and I bought tickets to São Paulo for Bruna and me. My grandfather bought his, Lúcia—my father's good friend and our teacher at the Batel school—also bought hers, along with other friends. But the wedding day never happened. My father and Daniela broke up, calling off the marriage just a week before the ceremony. I never understood why, but I also didn't want to pry, and he never told me the reason.

The healing aspect of my relationship with Daniela was very important. She, a very docile person, made me create a moment of internal calm and lucidity. It was healing to get out of the toxic relationship, into one filled with lightness. Her personality is very different from mine, and very different from Luciana's. So I did things that I wouldn't usually do and I don't normally do. I learned, in a way, from her, to enjoy a holiday, stay out of work on the weekend, consider vacations.

I came to São Paulo mostly to reduce the impact of international travel. It was a time when I was going to Canada and the United States a lot, and to Europe a little bit. It cost me a lot, you know? It created physical wear and tear as well. I started to stay more in São Paulo, instead of returning to Curitiba. I didn't even intend to settle here, although there was some desire. But I have never taken action in this direction.

I think the relationship was very good for me, and for her too. And for Ravi, who had another female presence in his life, with lightness, for the few years that our relationship lasted. But I understand that it was also very good that it ended. It would have been, professionally, a source of conflict.

Ravi:

While the wedding for Daniela and my father never happened, what happened afterward in São Paulo, was another great blessing in my father's life: Alissa. She gives him the space to continue creating and developing. They have managed to build a fantastic relationship that is positive for both of them.

I see in him a unique admiration for her, something I had never seen before. Today, he has this woman who inspires him, a woman who has changed him significantly. She provides him with family, structure, and routine.

I spent more time in São Paulo, no longer teaching in Curitiba. On the eve of a new course, I ended my relationship with Daniela. The next day, Alissa showed up, brought by a friend. She had never taken a class in the method and was unfamiliar with it. She had recently separated, ending her marriage, and was in the process of organizing custody and weekend visits for her children.

In that first class, she relaxed so much that she fell asleep on the yoga mat. I had to wake her up at the end of the class, which I found quite curious. We spoke very little during the year she progressed through the course. At the end of the course, she attended an international event of mine in Amsterdam with some friends. It was there that we began to talk more, and eventually, we started dating.

Alissa's personality was a big surprise to me. She is an intriguing mix of intelligence, family values, and citizenship values. She doesn't even seem Brazilian sometimes. She never parks crookedly in public parking lots and never invades another person's spot. She believes in doing the right thing and caring about others.

She is a very talented executive with an astute mind for business, which greatly fascinates me. Together, we undertook the opening of Kaiut Yoga Ateliê in São Paulo. We collaborated as a couple. All the technical and administrative aspects, the business model— those are entirely her domain. She essentially manages the space, so I can focus on what I do best, which is producing knowledge and teaching. It is not just a commercial partnership but a family venture, where she also talks with Ravi each week, guiding him in expanding the business.

Did the fact that she already had two children scare me?

I never saw children as a problem. At the beginning of our relationship, perhaps due to my past experiences, I was very reserved around them. But then the younger one, Felipo, broke the ice. Later, the older one, Prieta also warmed up to me. Their personalities gradually made me melt.

Nowadays, within the scope of my role, I am quite paternal with them. I have a consistent presence and participate in many aspects of their daily life and education.

Alissa:

My youngest was two years old, and my oldest was six when I separated in 2018. I spent a year trying to figure things out. I hadn't expected this to happen to me. It was very impactful.

At the time, I was in São Paulo, working at Restoque, one of the largest high-end fashion retail companies. The company had a portfolio of eight brands, including Le Lis, John John, Bo.Bô, Rosa Chá, and Dudalina. I was the commercial director of purchasing and planning and really liked what I did, working a lot. Prior to that, I had a career in the financial market, which gave me a large network of professional contacts.

I don't generally like to talk too much, especially about my personal matters. However, after the separation, I needed someone to confide in. I called my friend Marina, who told me about a yoga class with a teacher named Daniela. Marina had started taking classes with her a month after my separation. She signed me up, picked up a scholarship and class materials for me at the school, but it took me a while to find a gap in my schedule to attend. I only went to classes sporadically, on Saturdays when I didn't have custody of the children.

Things went on like this for some time, then one day, Marina mentioned that she had met a great yoga teacher at Daniela´s school, but she hadn't taken any courses with him.

To this writer, Alissa exudes the grace of a ballerina, indeed she did dabble in many activities as a child, including ballet, piano, and gymnastics. However, what she truly enjoyed throughout her life was basketball, volleyball, futsal, and even soccer. But eventually, she turned to yoga with Francisco.

For a long time, Francisco was just the teacher with whom she barely spoke.

I immediately saw that Francisco had a wealth of knowledge and thought he was overqualified for what he was doing. I also noticed something odd about him: outside of class he kept a distance from the students, which many people attributed to arrogance, but this disappeared during class time.

In September 2019, I resigned from my job with the intention of taking a sabbatical. I then learned that Francisco was going to hold an event in Amsterdam, an intensive for teachers. My friends encouraged me to go along.

On the last night in the Netherlands, they insisted on having a dinner with him. I remember joking,

"Wow, a dinner with the teacher!"

It was surprising because many were too intimidated to approach him, given his somewhat distant demeanor. This was in stark contrast to his classroom presence, where he seemed like an entirely different person.

At that dinner, we had a deeper conversation than ever before. Upon returning to Brazil, we began dating. Soon after, the COVID-19 pandemic started, which drastically changed his work and brought him closer to my family. My parents adored him. He gave up his apartment in São Paulo, and with my parents' help, found a rental home in Campinas, about 100 kilometers [63 miles] away from São Paulo where we lived.

Embracing the digital age, Francisco began offering video classes. We converted my parents' TV room into a makeshift studio from which he live-streamed his first classes on Facebook. Eventually, he set up a more permanent studio in his rented house.

Around this time, yoga became a significant part of my life. The body awareness I cultivated in my practice began to influence all my relationships, imbuing my interactions with care, kindness, and affection, whether with children or at work.

We then decided to open a yoga studio together in São Paulo, later expanding to a school. Seeking stability, we opted to own our school. We discovered and renovated a space in the Pinheiros neighborhood, launching the school at the end of 2022 when in-person classes resumed. I became heavily involved in strategic planning for Ravi's business expansion, including two hours of weekly Zoom meetings to discuss finances and future strategies. Francisco remained in São Paulo, focusing on his teaching, content creation, and knowledge-sharing, while Ravi, based in Curitiba, managed brand expansion under his father's guidance.

What do I love most about Francisco?

Initially, I saw him only as a teacher. Distant, perhaps even a bit arrogant. But I admired his presence in the classroom, the way he moved, spoke, taught yoga, and transmitted his method. His approach is uniquely effective and difficult to replicate. There are aspects of his work that are truly his own. His method and dedication truly make a positive impact on people in a very special way.

However, what captivates me most is not his professional side. I didn't fall in love with the teacher, I fell in love with the man. What intrigued me about him as a person, even from afar in Amsterdam, was his authenticity.

Imagine someone who has experienced everything he wanted in life. Francisco visited many yoga schools but never fell into stereotypes. He incorporated and transformed only what worked for him. He didn't just invent a method. He created a life that is good for him and beneficial to many others. He has the courage to be unapologetically himself, for better or worse.

His defining trait isn't rigidity but adaptability. He allows himself to change and evolve. I see this in his current phase, just enjoying the comfort of a little corner of his house, not wanting to travel as much, living close to the school, and walking to work. He seems to cherish staying at home.

Francisco is a man of intense energy. In the classroom he channels this wonderfully, balancing his energetic intensity with a sense of purpose, much like a small ball of fire. But outside the classroom, this intensity can sometimes be hard to manage. It may manifest as anger or aggression, with words he later regrets. But this is what makes him human.

The other day, I told him he transforms himself when he gets very angry, just like Hulk, the Marvel hero of immense strength who turns green when outraged by injustice. I added,

"When you get like this, you need to retreat to your cave and process all this energy."

The cave is his studio. And when he does retreat, he comes back calmer, often playful and humorous.

Well, I think it's time for us to understand how this transformation from Hulk Francisco to Yoga Francisco came to be. It's time to delve into the depths of the alchemical fire of pain and challenges that gave rise to this method. Kaiut Yoga.

Just turn the page and come along.

9

Legs Up

It is a natural tendency of the human mind, shaped by how we cognitively process reality, to organize and categorize what we know throughout existence in conceptual boxes. We label the white-haired gentleman who has served us for years at our favorite restaurant as a "friendly waiter." We refer to our children's school as "Lara and Luís' school." While this approach can be simplistic and reductionist, it serves a practical purpose—it helps us navigate a complex and challenging world by focusing on what serves us and discarding what doesn't. Memory plays a key role in this process, linking images with meanings that define and identify things for us.

When you think of yoga, a particular cliché image might come to mind: a beautiful woman with an angelic smile, serene face, hands together in the "namaste" gesture. She sits on a yoga mat in a cross-legged pose with a perfectly aligned spine. Looking like an athlete-goddess from Greek mythology, she embodies a modern oasis of calm amid our hectic lives.

Francisco's yoga school in São Paulo, Ateliê, is its own oasis of calm. Located in the pleasant neighborhood of Pinheiros, the space is thoughtfully designed to provide an escape from the city's relentless pace. Here, you can distance yourself from São Paulo's daily stress, with the congested traffic on Rebouças Avenue just a hundred feet (30 meters) away. Once inside, tranquility replaces the urgency of the metropolis.

However, when one thinks of Kaiut Yoga, and the type of practitioner you'll find there, a different image to a Greek goddess might come to mind. In conventional yoga classes, students are predominantly female, with women often more engaged in activities related to the evolution of consciousness, self-knowledge, body sensitivity, emotional intelligence, well-being, and health. But at Kaiut Yoga, instead of a solitary man you may have pictured among a group of women quietly radiating *joie de vivre* and an unspoken reverence for the sacredness of life, you will find something quite different.

In today's class at Ateliê, there are five women and five men. Yes, you read that correctly—half the class is men! This is a notable and honorable representation for the male gender, indeed. Let's give men a little credit here. Kaiut Yoga isn't a place where the human species will falter due to male ignorance about what truly matters in life.

The Kaiut Yoga method has a unique way of bridging the gap, speaking to men in a language that resonates. It brings attention to themes that can sometimes feel distant or unfamiliar, such as the evolution of consciousness, the value of self-care, care for others, and care for the planet. These are universal paths, open to all, irrespective of gender.

As you pass through the burgundy curtain at the entrance, you step into a rectangular space with a light-colored wooden floor, flanked by white side walls and a mustard-yellow back wall. Charcoal colored mats, red bolsters emblazoned with a golden K, black nylon yoga straps, and individual name plaques await the evening's students. Some students are already here, mingling in the small lounge area where they chat with Francisco, drink water, or snack on apples and nut bars from a basket. A mini library offers books by classic yoga authors like Hermógenes and B.K.S. Iyengar, as well as works on Ayurvedic medicine and emerging health sciences, such as those by American chiropractor Joe Dispenza.

Your attention is inevitably drawn to the practice space itself, where women—described here as the futuristic antennas of our species—sit alongside pioneering men. Among them are a journalist, a psychotherapist, entrepreneurs, executives, retirees, and a writer, ranging in age from 37 to 81. These individuals seem to possess a quiet certainty about what they want from life. They wait for Francisco to begin the class, their relaxed postures forming a striking image—one that may linger as their first, and perhaps most profound, symbolic memory of this experience.

They aren't seated cross-legged in the familiar sukhasana. Instead, they are lying on their backs, each on their own mat, heads resting on bolsters. Some have hands clasped behind their heads, while others tuck them lightly under the edges of the bolster. The tops of their heads point toward the center of the room, their legs raised with heels resting against the white walls. Legs are straight, knees extended as much as each body allows, ankles together, and thighs gently turned inward. This common starting position, known as "legs up the wall," sets the tone for the class.

The scene leaves a striking impression, a vivid "click" that imprints itself indelibly in your memory. As Francisco's voice commands your attention, your body instinctively responds. Perhaps you notice discomfort in your toes—long dormant from unconscious misuse—now awakened, twitching with unexpected vigor, even cramping. Francisco gently guides you to stay with this sensation, encouraging you to embrace it rather than resist. At first, your mind wrestles with the seeming contradiction, but gradually, it begins to understand the counterintuitive logic that defines Kaiut Yoga.

Metaphorically, the method flips on its head the distorted logic of our consumerist and reductionist society—a world built on narrow, simplistic principles. It challenges the over-conditioned mind, gently nudging you beyond your comfort zone. In doing so, it dismantles ingrained paradigms, restoring awareness of the life force flowing through your feet and its vital connection to the health of your entire body.

Psychologically, the method offers respite for the nervous system—a chance to recover from the relentless strain imposed by a civilization often severed from natural wisdom. It reawakens the integrated intelligence of the mind, emotions, and body, enabling sustainable regeneration. This process activates health at the deepest levels of both consciousness and physiology, fostering a profound sense of harmony and well-being.

How did Francisco arrive at this profound understanding? How did he distill the organic and spontaneous logic underlying his method into these carefully designed positions and practices?

The creation and development of Kaiut Yoga was not a linear process, nor did it begin consciously—it unfolded in stages.

Following my experience in Italy, I decided that I would not mess with this yoga business anymore, because it was a bad thing. It had many gross flaws. There was mysticism, there was religion, there was an absence of technique, there were a lot of things that were wrong. So, I moved away, although tried to keep in touch with what was happening.

I came back very hurt, with a lot of chronic pain, caused by poor yoga technique. The injury to the hamstring muscles in both my legs would take me 10 years to heal.

Then, in England, while I went to study polarity therapy there was also supposedly a lot of good quality yoga, with many good teachers, most of them Indian, as the England-India connection is so strong. It was then I began to view yoga differently and identified patterns of injury associated with various yoga methods.

It was there that I realized I needed to forge my own path, guided by intuition. Thus, one root of the method lay in the knowledge from ancestral yoga, polarity therapy, and new health approaches that attracted me. The other was in observing patterns of pain in others and myself.

However, upon returning from Europe, I primarily worked in chiropractic, relegating yoga to a hobby and conducting experimental small-group practices.

When I accepted Theresa's invitation to go to New York—who had seen my experimental classes in Curitiba where my method was forming—I felt something promising was happening, but I was a little uncertain about it. There were no other references for comparison.

On a Sunday morning amidst a blizzard, I held my first class at her studio. Seventy people attended, all experienced with various yoga teachings. I had never taught such a large group before. To be immediately accepted and recognized by those knowledgeable practitioners was incredibly affirming. I understood then that what I was doing was really good. This outline of the method had its own dynamics, effectively fostering body awareness.

I spent several months there. Despite Theresa's talk of getting me a residence visa and hiring me as a permanent teacher, similar to what she had done with many Indian teachers, I was not attracted by it. I never had the desire to leave Brazil, as travel inherently lacks pleasure for me.

I came back to Brazil because I wanted to do excellent work, but at home. Upon returning, I began offering regular yoga classes and soon had around 80 dedicated students. My focus had shifted towards using yoga to impact health, performance, and longevity in the long term. I realized I did not want to be a chiropractor for the rest of my life, and the idea of returning to clinical work no longer appealed to me. I started thinking about yoga from a systemic perspective and its long-term benefits.

I began to better elaborate the preparation of my yoga classes. Naturally, I had drawn inspiration from watching my parents meticulously prepare their classes at home. My dad, in particular, approached class preparation with a theatrical flair. This influenced my habit of drawing and scribbling class outlines everywhere, on napkins, on the dining table. However, this time, I knew I needed to refine my process.

I was still seeing the occasional chiropractic client when, one day, one of them missed an appointment. Seizing the free time, I went to the yoga room to take a breather and sat on the floor.

The cleaning woman entered the room and asked how I wanted her to set up the room. This question, as simple as it was, sparked an important realization: the room itself is a primary piece of equipment in the method. This subtle shift in perspective became the foundation for further refining my approach.

The most important insight I had was that the student needs to feel warmly welcomed. If students do not feel welcomed, they tend to control the environment. However, if they are well received, they enter a passive emotional and neurological state that allows for an appropriate internal positioning and processing speed conducive to practice.

I was sitting on the floor, surrounded by mats. From my position, I saw them from a different angle. I asked the cleaning woman to put the mats down at a 90-degree angle to the wall. As I watched, it struck me that the mats seemed to rise from the floor, resembling a chiropractic table, before returning to the ground.

That moment completely changed my view on what I was doing. It revolutionized my understanding of the purpose behind my actions. The previous boundaries vanished. I realized that every yoga mat could be a chiropractic table, and every yoga position a joint manipulation. Everything began to take on a new design.

This experience, for me, marks the true birth of the method.

You know when water is heating up in the kettle, you hardly notice it until it suddenly boils, ready for your tea? Or how a seed quietly germinates beneath the soil, hidden from view, only to surprise you when a delicate plant breaks through the surface into the sunlight?

The vision of the mats at the wall was like this—a sudden, powerful blossoming. It was the culmination of something that had been germinating for a long time, silently taking root beneath the surface; growth driven by the search for light on the surface... the pain...

I had some incidents with my knees that caused me to experience pain that was very limiting. My knees wouldn't bend, stretch, or move. During a busy period in my chiropractic work, the pain would accumulate and hit me all at once after I got home from my last client on Friday. It was a comprehensive pain that affected not only my knees but also my feet, fascia, and entire muscle chains throughout my legs.

I had to lie in bed, in a dark room, from Friday to Saturday, as there was nothing else I could do to alleviate the knee pain. I had to stay still and wait for the pain to subside by Sunday or Monday morning, at which point I would muster the energy to return to work. By the following Friday, the pain would return in a relentless, cyclical crisis.

I began to realize that I needed to rescue my joints. Physical therapy, manipulation, and other treatments seemed irrelevant or totally inefficient. Various doctors offered surgical solutions, but I was increasingly aware that many of these surgeries often ended in failure.

I started gaining a better understanding of what "rescue" meant. I was mapping out pathways, knowing they had to address the pain directly. I started with focused work on the feet and hips, I did this by entering the pain, provoking the pain, activating a healing stimulus within the pain.

Nothing else had worked. Conventional methods had failed to deliver results. I realized I had to look within. This led to an understanding that in going to the pain, you are not causing the problem, right? Going into the pain is about provoking the solution, and the solution lies within the problem itself.

Once an injury occurs, you can't separate yourself from the pain. There's no way you can say, "my knee hurts." Your knee doesn't hurt. There's something causing the knee to hurt. The source of the pain resides within, but the knee itself is not the pain.

As human beings, we often display a profound tendency towards overidentification, driven by a strong ego that leads us to identify more than is necessary with our physical bodies. The restrictions in movement we experience are not inherent to our bodies but are imposed upon our bodies over decades. This insight is what gives rise to the method. The method gives the student enough understanding of this process to shift from identifying with the problem, to identifying with the solution.

Initially, it is essential to approach sensations conservatively to establish a genuine sense of safety, so you are not trapped by defense mechanisms that block the process. This is not work done by [students] Ed, Sol, Frances, and Gregório, and their individual personalities. Instead, it is something that happens from the natural intelligence that lies beyond an individual's personality. This is the focus of the method.

Each position in Kaiut Yoga has an essential element. I developed the method one step at a time. The method has to do with processes that involve a lot of awareness and requires acceptance of reality. Because you can't transform what you don't accept. And you don't accept what you don't understand. Thus, the method is also a place for understanding certain processes in nature.

Did I encounter the reactive mechanism of non-acceptance of pain in my own personal process when I was developing me method?

Indeed! I experienced the emotion of anger!

However, the relationship between anger and pain did not dissolve concurrently with the transformation of pain. These things do not dismantle simultaneously. First, the physical structure changes, which then leads to a deeper understanding that everything is subject to change. This realization becomes a tangible entry point into another realm, which is the transformation within the emotional field.

Over the years, I have observed many individuals, particularly men with significant physical issues, who have changed their patterns of thought, behavior, and even personality. In my own experience, I noticed that mental rigidity and emotional reactivity, characteristic of a somewhat hot-headed temperament, gradually softened and dissipated.

As you journey through Francisco's creative process, you might begin to piece together what the method truly is. Perhaps you've already formed a symbolic image that encapsulates the essence of Kaiut Yoga. Yet, you might still crave a clearer, more conceptual synthesis. If your mind is inclined toward concrete, structured thinking—as so many of us are—you might think, "Ah, I get it... The method is the organized sequence of classes... It's the set of positions, like those distinctive poses with legs up the wall, the practitioners lying on their backs, heads resting on bolsters..."

Well, quietly... just between us... can I suggest something? Hasty conclusions may not be the best approach here. An intricate tangle of paths led to the method. It was carefully dismantled, recombined, and refined through various means over time before blossoming into its current form.

There is no shortcut to understanding. You will arrive there, but at a slow, evolutionary pace. Thought and feeling must gradually build towards their apex, culminating in a sudden burst of clarity and integration. It's like a radiant flash at the dawn of your search, illuminating the indigo sky.

The method has reached a point of maturity—it is in a very sustainable and coherent place. It is grounded in its founding logic, its intrinsic essence. This foundational basis arises from my analysis of the Vedas, the ancient body of knowledge from Hindu civilization. Within the Vedas, much of Ayurvedic medicine is intertwined with ancestral yoga. In this context, I discovered a brilliant phrase: "give back to the human being his nature."

This phrase redefines yoga, distinguishing it from much of what we see today. It inspired me to seek out all fragments of yoga that proposed a return to this natural pattern. Fifteen to twenty thousand years ago, homo sapiens bent forward hundreds of times a day to pick things up from the ground. This frequent use created a favorable condition.

This ancient homo sapien didn't bend his knees, drop his hips, or contract his abdomen to reach the ground. He simply extended his straight spine, stretched out his arm and hand, and took the fruit or root to eat, whatever. There was no joint degeneration. There are ancient bones that show no signs of degenerative joint disease. This guy, who squatted to have a bowel movement, had no lumbar degeneration.

Today, it is very rare to find an adult human being without some degree of joint, hip, or spine degeneration. When I started analyzing this, I thought, "damn it, wait a second! All my clinic patients experience lumbar crises when they pick something up off the floor."

I began to view the postures of ancestral yoga with new eyes. I started to ask myself, what is the essence of a yoga position? The essence is a natural pattern. I came to understand that there was a form of yoga that existed even before the birth of Ayurveda. The Vedas were speaking to the need to rescue this pre-Vedic human nature, predicting that one day humanity would lose its natural essence and break away from its roots.

That's the reality we face today. Human beings often feel disconnected from nature. However, the most brilliant idea that ancestral yoga offers us is the possibility of reconnection. The human body is intrinsically linked to nature itself. This is the most extraordinary aspect of human development. No matter how sophisticated civilization becomes—regardless of one's attire, apartment, environment, or car—we remain human bodies, a collective of microbiomes coexisting. Yoga emerged from a visionary understanding, from someone who foresaw this moment and began to design a solution.

We are an ever-evolving planet, and an evolving, highly adaptable species. The conditions that shaped homo sapiens on the African savannah were different from those they encountered as they expanded to Asia and other parts of the planet. Likewise, the conditions of our time are different.

The natural context that once generated a bromeliad plant in the Atlantic Forest of Brazil is the same that allows the City of São Paulo to plant bromeliads in urban gardens today. Cities represent a new form of nature, an evolving environment adapting to more inclusive urban spaces. The natural environment will never obstruct Nature, as cities are a part of it.

From that point, I understood the importance of rescuing the roots of ancestral yoga while also recognizing the need to adapt and adjust postures to suit contemporary conditions. This led to the creation of new postures in the development of Kaiut Yoga. The aim is to stimulate adaptability for movement and mobility that society has put to sleep.

The method is an exercise in reclaiming ancestry. It is the revival of an expression of Nature. This rescue sets natural mechanisms in motion, allowing Nature itself to create a therapeutic process. The tools, positions, and approach to classes help the student to stop thinking, enabling Nature to take over. The method incorporates asymmetrical and unpredictable stimuli, avoiding specialization but fostering a high degree of resilience. The method is a place that rescues our inner Nature.

When Nature takes control, there is no negativity. Modern human beings, from a false sense of security and predictability, often assume the worst possible outcome when faced with a seemingly insurmountable challenge. Modern human beings have this strong tendency to lean towards the negative.

Yet Nature operates in a state of equilibrium—a state that is mildly positive, neither anxious nor destructive to the point of generating negativity. Consider a stray dog. It may be hungry, but it doesn't anxiously tear into the next garbage bag, worried it might find nothing. It simply keeps moving forward.

That is why I say that Kaiut Yoga cultivates a chronic state of presence with emotional coherence. Emotional coherence is the state where all of Nature operates harmoniously, much like the bromeliads thriving in the flowerbeds of Haddock Lobo Street near Paulista Avenue, this top iconic venue in our largest metropolis in South America...

Wow! What a fantastic journey—revealing the fundamentals and historical context of the method. However, it only hints at another ultra-significant transformation—one symbolized by the sight of the mats against the wall, and consequently the legs up the wall pose. This was a pivotal moment when Francisco began to see his work through completely new eyes. He realized that his life's purpose had shifted from being solely a clinical curator to something far more complex and distinctive. The curator role still existed but had evolved into a unique form.

Instead of viewing clinical work as an exercise in surrender, I came to realize that teaching offers the greatest contribution one can make to the planet. Teaching is the truest form of service in the most spiritual sense of the word. Serving others through education holds the value of a kind of priesthood, as it is a service without subservience. It bears spiritual significance. This service delivers positive change and creates a wave of systemic impact. Nothing is more crucial for the betterment of our little planet than education.

Do you agree? Disagree? I can't know your opinion on this. However, you can know for sure that this is Francisco's truth.

You can understand that it is from this point on that his mission as an educator truly begins, marked by the launch of his first teacher training program. I can sense your curiosity about how the method developed in practice from that eureka moment involving legs up the wall.

From that moment on, remarkable cases began to emerge, consolidating the method's results. Additionally, real-life personalities from this Brazilian epic of international reach begin to add their voices to the narrative.

Before we move on, a comment on the euphoric expression "eureka." This expression, that comes from an ancient Greek legend, is used to describe a sudden, important discovery. The wise scientist-philosopher Archimedes was commissioned by King Hiero to solve a complicated problem. It's worth noting that the concept of science as we understand it today may not have existed in antiquity, when areas of knowledge were not yet specialized; science and philosophy may have been a unified, integrated way of knowing. Anyway, Archimedes, was sitting in a bathtub when the solution came to him. So excited—or perhaps relieved given his neck might have been on the line—he ran out into the streets naked, shouting... "Eureka!"

Now we can move forward with this increasingly fascinating story—Francisco's, not Archimedes'. And here we cross a checkpoint, stepping forward through new narrative gates.

10

The Empty Spot and a Code Beyond Pain

I began referring to my original school, where I conducted experimental classes, as a laboratory—it was where I had my first experiences with students and with therapeutic issues that contributed to the development of the method. These classes started in 1999 in a rented space in Alto da Rua XV, a quiet neighborhood in Curitiba, yet famous for its nightlife. From there, I moved as the number of students grew, and I opened new classes. First, I moved the school to another place in the Botanical Garden and then a third place, in Praça da Espanha, in the Batel neighborhood, until I transferred to another house a few meters from that first building, right there in the square.

It was operating within this laboratory mindset and atmosphere that gave me the chance to develop an especially important skill for delivering the method: the ability to identify patterns of behavior, patterns in the body, in the joints, and in the movements of individuals experiencing pain. Over time, I also discovered that patterns are not just something to observe—they can be created and used strategically to facilitate healing and transformation. Little by little, I learned how to work with these patterns to my advantage, shaping the foundation of the method itself.

In a classroom with 30 people, I see 60 knees, and each knee is unique. There is no rule or protocol for dealing with the knee. There is a unique solution for each knee. While the person is usually looking for a rule to deal with their problem, the method offers a search for a solution. This requires a lot of creativity. The specific technique to be applied is born from finding the student's needs, in a highly creative process.

All patterns are important, and they emerge in micromovements. Recognizing these patterns is foundational to the method. It was from there that I designed the 100 foundational class plans of the method. Their function is to offer a kind of x-ray of the student's whole body and their patterns of behavior, emotional reactivity, and nervous system. The classes are a great diagnostic process.

Who is this human being, the student? How do they move? How do they behave in a classroom environment? How do they react to blind and unknown spots in their body? How do they respond to pain? How do they receive information and feedback about themselves? How long does it take for them to open to the therapeutic process?

The classes are structured so that the teacher can masterfully present the method to the student while also giving the teacher the opportunity to collect an immense volume of information on an individual. Teachers are trying to understand things like: What is the relationship between the student's mental attitude and the patterns of self-sabotage? What defense mechanisms arise—against movement, against the voluntary awareness of pain, or against approaching the body from an angle that they are not used to?

This is where I formulated a guiding principle of the method: the student needs to fall in love with the result. For the student to fall in love with the result, the teacher has only one opportunity, which is the first class. In this first class, the teacher needs to enchant the student while remaining firmly grounded in ethical practice.

The "enchantment class" is one in which the student falls in love with the process and the possibility of the result. To do this, the teacher needs to read the student instantly, without any judgment or prejudice. The teacher needs to find the language that addresses the listener's needs.

In a class, you don't deliver results. You deliver sensations and perspective. When the student falls in love and comes back for the second class, then you have the opportunity to build towards something more. The ultimate goal is for the student to be linked to the practice and process for the rest of their life, working on changing their biomechanical, energetic, psychological system.

A method is a language. Every language has its own grammar, which consists of the signs and elements that compose it, as well as the codes and rules of combination that make it function, all based on its intrinsic logic. When a new language is created and emerges with a very distinct and innovative identity, the creator faces a unique challenge.

What challenged me the most in the development of Kaiut Yoga was allowing myself the creative freedom to think independently.

This independent thinking must originate somewhere. Fortunately, we all have a history behind us. Collective history, as well as personal history, leaves its mark on each of us. In my case, being Brazilian, receiving an incredible education, having parents who were teachers, and experiencing moments of enchantment have all influenced me. Even so, few things truly prepare us to think independently. It is exceedingly difficult to discern which elements of collective history and individual experiences have real value and which need to be discarded in your creative process.

In the first few years of analyzing yoga methods, I understood that many people were doing things that seemed to be right but were in fact wrong. What was wrong was not the position in yoga. It was how a given posture was being approached and used.

I began to deconstruct everything, in a sense. It was as if each position were a puzzle of a thousand pieces. I found that the problem lay in traditional yoga methods wanting to somehow subdue the student or the body to fit into a position. I came to understand that each student has their ideal and healing version of each position.

The question shifted. It was no longer about the student conforming to a position. Instead, it became about the student embodying a position, like wearing a tailor-made garment.

There's a sense of perfection, of fit, that's always unique. Always, always. Therefore, I do not rename the positions, as they have been named for hundreds of years. However, the names could have contributed to a better understanding and use. There have been rare moments in the history of yoga when the positions were used exceptionally well, becoming enduring therapeutic resources. The position is a guiding star, like the North Star or the Southern Cross. It sets the direction. But the process of getting there... that's the true art.

This is distinctive first element of Kaiut Yoga. While everyone in the yoga world focuses on building positions, I aim to deconstruct them. Everyone wants to force bodies into standardized positions in the world of yoga. I want to deconstruct the rigidity of the body, so that the position can be born on its own. From the concept of unlocking and restoring functions, I created what I call "fragments." These are fragments of a process that will eventually come together to form a future position.

An alphabet. A code. For those of you who already practice and want to continue, go practice after reading this real-life story. For those who engage symbolically with this narrative, journey on. We all find signs on a map, but which direction do they point?

The classic yoga positions inspire these fragments, but they need to be translated for today's humans—for those who don't kneel on the ground, for those who don't squat for their intestines to function, and for those who don't sit around the campfire.

I understood that what hurt people was not the classical positions themselves, but the absence of basic functionality of modern humans. The reality is that someone may feel fit and healthy, engaging in regular physical activities and adhering to contemporary fitness ideals. However, their body is often shaped by aesthetic standards and a narrow understanding of health. Despite their perceived fitness, they may find themselves unable to kneel on the ground. Our ancestral functionality is lost.

Just today, I was talking to a student who has already had two shoulder surgeries and is scheduled to have shoulder prosthesis at some point. I was preoccupied with the issue and felt compelled to explain,

"Lígia, you've never had a shoulder problem."

Her shoulders suffered, her shoulders hurt, and the ligaments ruptured. But the problem was never the shoulders.

"You had a postural change that has to do with your life history, profession, and personality. This change in your spine is what caused your shoulder pain. Medicine has spent your entire life treating the symptom. If you were to get the prosthesis, it would cause a significant debilitating shock to your system, but no one would be addressing the actual cause. "

We've lost connection with this ancestral functionality, so I sought it out. I looked for the positions that everyone overlooked and then looked for the initial steps of each one, because I believed that's where the gap was. The empty spot.

When you reflect on this chapter concerning the development of the method, you find Francisco, the scientist, in the original and pure sense of the word. A scientist who researches, analyzes, and seeks out existing knowledge but also explores its voids, setting up hypotheses for solutions. He tests them. His gaze is not limited to minute details in isolation, which is the pitfall of many researchers, excessively conditioned by super specialization that fragments reality, causing them to lose sight of the whole. Francisco is not interested in solitary facts. Because he is a pattern hunter.

The path to the method involved much observation of other yoga teachers too. I observed openly, without judgment, as if I were a scanner. Scanning mentally, I could see what was not harmonious in a yoga position. It was as if I were using a microscope, but instead of the lens showing me a fixed sample of something material, it revealed patterns. Then, I generated questions, created multiple scenarios of possibilities, theories, and theses, and finally drew my conclusions.

I realized that virtually all of the great yogis of this era had an overloaded nervous system, characterized by tension, anxiety, and irritability. Hence, the need to develop what I call "opening rituals", which are exercises designed to regulate the autonomic nervous system.

Many people come to take classes every day, choosing yoga as a way to relieve stress. However, they actually need to relieve their stress before they can fully engage in yoga. So, I created a mechanism to discharge the person's nervous system before class begins. This allows them to have a more in-depth experience. I can accommodate all individuals, regardless of their backgrounds. Say, there are three individuals that come to class—a entrepreneur, a senior executive, and a young executive—they have just left the office and are all highly stressed.

What do I do with them?

First, I establish a safety mechanism. I guide all three individuals, who are operating predominantly from their sympathetic nervous system, into a parasympathetic mode of operation, which prioritizes cellular nutrition and rejuvenation. I don't push them to approach yoga positions in a performative manner. Instead, I just tell them to immerse themselves inside the position. This approach calls for self-responsibility and maturity, because I challenge everyone to deal with enormous levels of sensation. However, I emphasis this is not to be done aggressively or competitively.

Oh, a moment, please! Just a short pause, right now. In case you forgot, or maybe you didn't pay much attention in that biology or anatomy class in high school... Here's a quick reminder about the nervous system.

The nervous system is this intricate network of neural tissues that orchestrates the body's functions. It acts as a highly sophisticated electrical and chemical power plant, an advanced communication network, a motor control center, and a vast database. It governs everything from the muscle movements that enable walking to the emotional responses elicited by joy or sadness. Additionally, it regulates the heartbeat and blood pressure, is key to the complex processes of memory formation, and controls the responses to sexual arousal. This remarkable system, born from the enigma of human life, underpins every aspect of our existence.

One integral part of the nervous system is the autonomic nervous system (ANS), which oversees the functioning of internal organs such as the stomach, heart, and kidneys, among others. This system is further divided into two other systems—more aptly called subsystems from a systemic perspective—the sympathetic and the parasympathetic nervous systems. The sympathetic subsystem stimulates bodily processes, while the parasympathetic subsystem inhibits them.

Nature operates within a vital rhythm and thrives within a dynamic range of equilibrium of these subsystems. However, our modern, stress-filled, urbanized civilization, disrupts this natural rhythm. The sympathetic nervous system is chronically overactivated, keeping the body in a perpetual state of fight or flight in response to constant pressures and demands. Conversely, the parasympathetic system acts as a natural antidote to its twin, conserving, restoring, and regenerating tissues. For the body to function optimally, it needs to be guided back into a state of calm.

This is the context within which the method operates—offering a pathway to recalibrate the nervous system and reconnect with the body's inherent intelligence.

The opening ritual is the sole moment in which we condition the student within the method. But what exactly is this ritual?

You've seen it. The executive who arrived a few minutes early for class, coming straight from work. She only greeted us and a few peers before heading into the practice room. She lay on her yoga mat, legs up against the wall, and head on the bolster.

She's already had the experience, and it's this experience that pulls her back into the room after a busy day at the office. She returns because she has identified results, perhaps even unconsciously, and seeks to replicate them. Behind every personality lies intelligence, and when you communicate with this intelligence using natural positive reinforcement, the person doesn't get caught in these places of "Oh, I don't have discipline... I lack body awareness..." I don't think the person has to be disciplined. People need to understand the result and the consistency of the result they get. And remember, it is not the teacher who delivers results.

When the person comes into contact with their pain, there is an intelligence that perceives the purpose of the rescue. Then, the person no longer identifies with the pain and does not identify with the difficulty or the disability. He identifies with the possibility of rescue. It is remarkably interesting to observe that when the work is delivered with the correct language, it does not trigger defense mechanisms, and it does activate the personality. It goes straight through these layers. It goes to a natural and ancestral intelligence that is behind everything. And to a place where the student understands the deep meaning of the work.

I also understood the importance of using correct language and creating a one hundred percent safe environment. This realization marked a significant improvement in the quality of the classes and the development of the method. That's why I embraced simplicity. Lying on the floor, on the mat, with legs up against the wall, letting gravity do its work. I realized that I could operate with a degree of physical demand on the body and joints while also applying pressure on the mind and emotions. The more pressure applied, the greater the results and better connection with intelligence would emerge.

The ritual, the practice, the positions, the nervous system response, everything in this process leads me to assert that this method is not just a yoga activity but a hygiene habit. Practicing Kaiut Yoga is more akin to flossing than engaging in physical exercise. You sanitize every joint and every system in your body. Once cleansing is complete, you begin to unlock your potential. As this potential is rescued, you can then start to expand it.

A crucial aspect of the method is that it is one hundred percent a sanitization process, in the most literal sense. Nervous system hygiene and circulatory hygiene. When joints are underutilized, chemical depositions, the waste from the body, build up. When you start to engage in the process of rescuing those joints, you bring the body back to regular use.

Regular for whom? For the orthopedist? No, regular for the human species. Once the rescue is complete and potential has been expanded, the method offers what I call evolutionary work. This is work that progresses to another level of results, surpassing even what we consider normal today.

Evolution of the species, evolution of the individual, expansion of consciousness, overcoming limits, and the qualitative development of the human being toward its untapped potential—these are the themes that are at the core of the method. They are implicit in Francisco's speech and certainly spark curiosity and a sense of possibility within this story. Yet, before we move forward to understand how the method bridges these profound ideas, all uniquely centered on body awareness, it's worth stepping back for a moment. Let's shift our perspective to illuminate the scenario in front of us.

In the ancient cultures of humanity and the living traditions of indigenous peoples, the figure of the healing shaman occupies a special place. These individuals possess a rare ability to navigate the subtle dimensions of existence while remaining firmly grounded in the concrete aspects of life. They act as conduits for the life forces that sustain health, bridging the seen and unseen. This archetypal role is timeless, continually adapting to the unique conditions of each era and culture.

In contemporary global society, the archetype of the shaman has evolved, emerging as modern healers who embody the intuitive sensitivity to natural processes alongside scientifically validated knowledge. These healers blend ancient wisdom with contemporary rigor, applying insights that have been tested and proven in controlled settings while retaining the essence of their ancestral roots.

An important link between the traditional shaman and the modern healer lies in their authority within their communities. It is not merely the result of their sharp discernment of others or their mastery of their craft through deep study. Often, their credibility is profoundly linked to their own personal journey—a transformative experience of confronting and overcoming a significant health challenge. This intimate understanding of healing becomes the foundation for their work, creating a bridge between their inner path and the service they offer to others.

The last major crisis I faced with my knees occurred when I put my daughter, Malu, on my shoulders for a walk. I had previously endured a severe knee problem caused by yoga, which I eventually resolved without any medical intervention. However, after that day's walk, the pain in my knees returned with a vengeance. It was a horrible crisis. Everything seemed to go wrong, leading to many months of intense pain.

Walking in the classroom hurt a lot. I also attended to many people, and I had to kneel. The feeling of pain radiated widely throughout my body. It took me to an emotionally complex place.

I vividly remember one day sitting on the edge of the bed, trying to figure out where to begin the rescue. Everything felt utterly rotten, literally decomposed. I dropped my feet to the floor, turned my toes upside down, and pressed them against the ground. I discovered a layer of stiffness at the base of my toes, across the tops, and along the instep. This stiffness involved intense local pain, but it didn't feel like the wrong kind of pain; it felt like a necessary pain. Even if it wasn't, I needed to test it, because my condition was so extreme.

I began experimenting. At first, I tried on the floor, but the pain was too intense, so I moved back to the bed. I found positions that allowed me to isolate the pain, working only on my toes, first on one foot, then the other. Gradually, I noticed a change in my knees. It was as though I was rescuing something, in crossing through this particular pain, which didn't hurt in the usual sense. I continued to explore what I could do, how I could do it, and how far I could push myself. A few weeks later, I was able to bend my knees. From that point, they continuously improved. When the pain was over, I entered a cycle of discovering the potential of movement.

As you already know, this incident was neither the first nor the last involving my knees. In the future, there would even issues that would seem ordinary, were it not for the painful outcomes.

When Ravi was born, I tried to return to a martial art that I had practiced as a teenager. At the end of the first class, after everyone had left following post-class conversation circle, I decided to take advantage of being in the space to practice some yoga positions. As I move into the lotus position, I heard a distinct "pleck!" I didn't pay much attention because I felt nothing. However, hours later at home, the pain arrived. And it was insane!

This time, I thought I had cracked a bone, really. I rushed to the hospital, and they did an X-ray. The doctor came to explain,

"It's a fracture. It will have to be plastered. You'll have to wear a brace."

I didn't even argue, I just said,

"Okay, okay."

They directed me to another waiting room, where they would call me for the procedure. However, as soon as the doctor had exited the area, I just got up and left.

Francisco remembered that he could rely on his own path of rescue. He recalled the past incident that had been resolved through natural means, on the physical plane, before the creation of the method. This case provided important lessons that would later be channeled into the method.

With the first major knee problem I had before Malu was born, the frustration of not being able to heal, at first, brought me anger, a lot of anger. And hopelessness. From this hopelessness came a very strong depression. I became depressed to the point of not wanting to leave the house, not wanting to go to work, and once lying on the bathroom floor. Because I didn't see the point in anything. It all had to do with the intense and unrelenting pain, which continued even when the depression passed.

Why the pain continued? I don't know. My impression is that something in my system decided to look for a solution. I was accommodating, adapting to the pain. I didn't have as much understanding of the body, nor did I have any idea that so much pain could be relieved with a yoga position. When new medical tests proved that the fracture had consolidated, I looked for a natural resource to cure the pain by myself.

I found the shiatsu work of the Japanese physician Katsusuke Serizawa, author of Tsubo: Vital Points for Oriental Therapy. Serizawa's work was very relevant to the method in the late 1990s. I pulled from the book techniques that I applied myself. To my surprise, I came out of the pain crisis. It was a relief, even though there remained a residual pain. But the knees remained dysfunctional. They could not handle my workload. Exhaustion came very quickly.

While I was in strong pain, I also became angrier, to the point that I broke things. I remember once breaking a chair. I was alone in the room, in a lot of pain, and I needed to vent somehow. Little by little, I realized that anger simply did not bring any positive or at least minimally positive results. When I saw this, hopelessness came.

But what good did all this bringing me? And how would this be reflected in my work and the method?

From such experiences I gained an enormous ability to understand the pain of others—a deep capacity for empathy. I learned how to very quickly make an individual feel heard and understood in their pain, through non-verbal communication and through knowing what to hear and what not to hear. It meant I could be very empathetic with very few words.

However, I also understood one of my students' main complaints in the beginning: that I delivered results but spoke little and explained almost nothing. I saw that there was a void there and that I needed to develop verbal skills as well.

I understood that I needed this resource. I committed myself to reading one book a week, often two. I read many books on teaching techniques, personal development, neuroscience, and new attitudes in health. I always chose authors with great verbal communication skills.

Albino Tramontina, now 85 years old, was one of Francisco's first students in Curitiba and remains a regular attendee of the school in Batel. Over the years, he witnessed this evolution of the method and Francisco, yet he recognizes that Francisco's deep empathetic understanding of his students has remained constant from the beginning.

Businessman, partner, and active director of the company representing Unimed—a giant in the Brazilian health insurance sector, Albino continues to lead an active life. When this is being written, he still kicks a soccer ball around from time to time, a feat that he struggled to do 25 years ago.

The diagnosis pointed to a significant wear and tear of cartilage. It hurt a lot when my body cooled down after exercise. After playing soccer, I had to stay out for 15 days with a calf strain. The doctors were already indicating surgery for hip prosthesis, when they referred me to four massage sessions with Antonio. But he took a vacation, and then he recommended Francisco to me. And when Francisco started teaching yoga classes, first my wife Silvana enrolled, and soon started telling me that the practice was incredibly good, that I should go.

I postponed it a lot, but shortly after I started, my orthopedist said that I had not improved but had stabilized the situation. Gradually, I reached ninety to ninety-five percent pain free, a rate that I keep today. The pain that stays does not bother me to the point of prohibiting me from playing soccer.

Then, my three children came to do yoga with Francisco as well. I became friends with him. One of his standout qualities is how he conducts his classes. His voice carries a magnificent, firm command that leaves no room for misunderstanding—you always know exactly what he means. Add this to a lot of charisma, a lot of competence, and a remarkable ability to connect with people, and you have a truly sensational professional.

Sometimes, you're in the middle of a class with 40 students, and you feel tempted to ease up a bit because something is hurting or you're tired. But you'd better think twice before doing that. Because Francisco sees a lot. As he often says, "I know a lot about the body of each of you here." And then he gets on your case!

Did I have the surgery to get a hip prosthesis?
I never needed it.

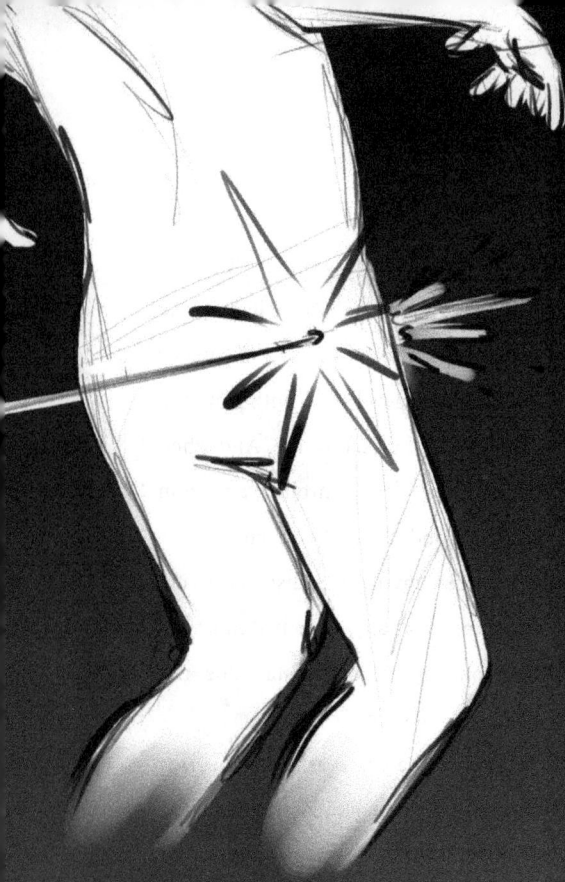

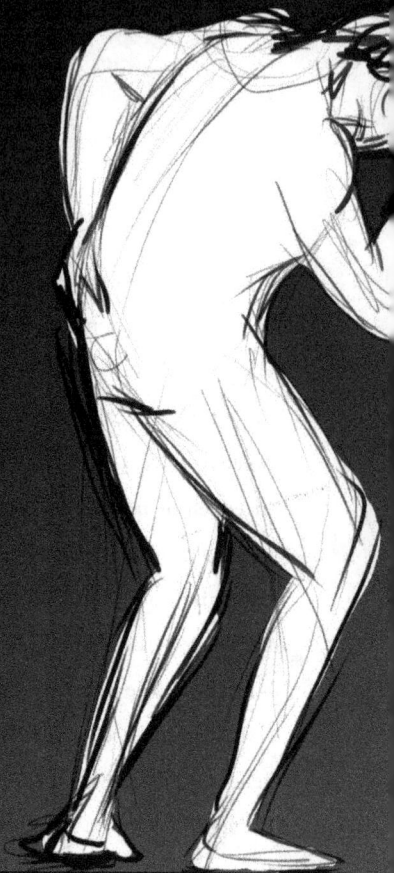

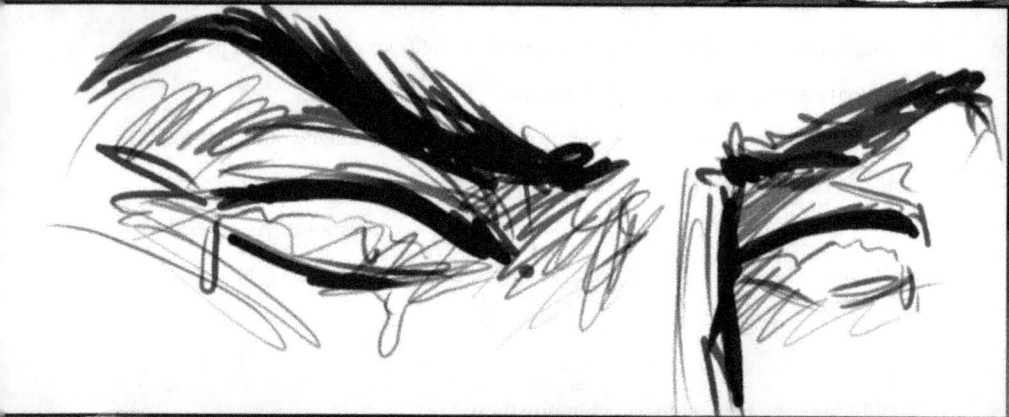

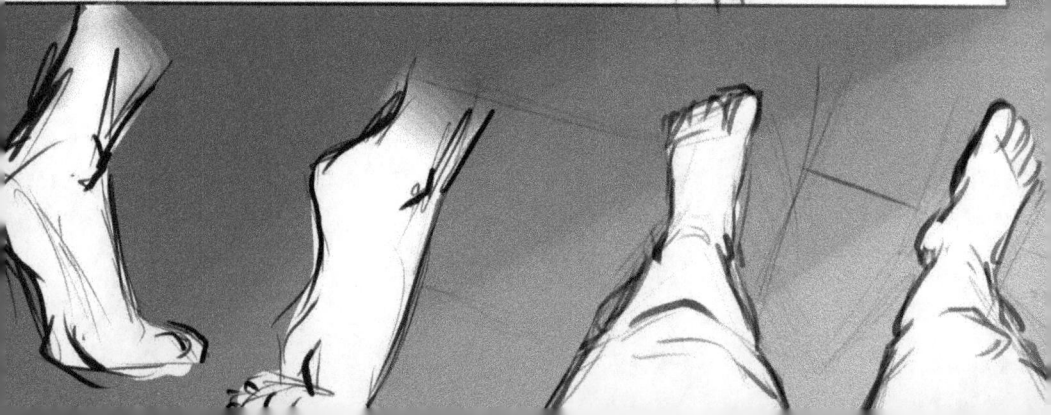

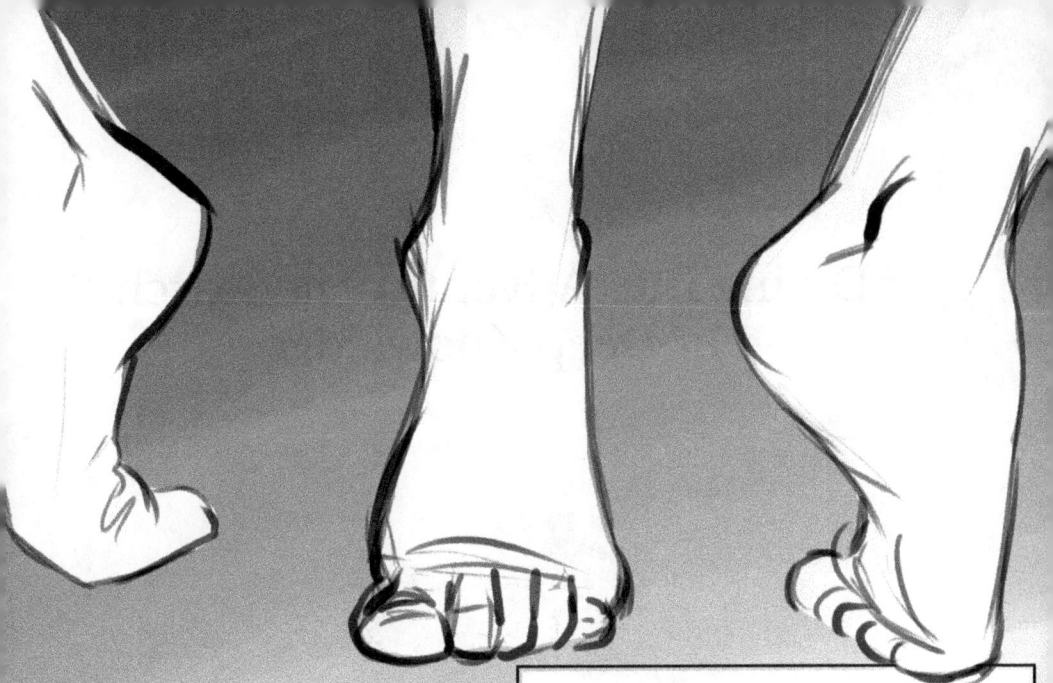

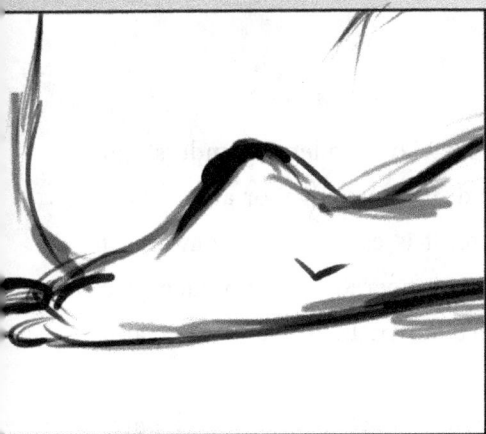

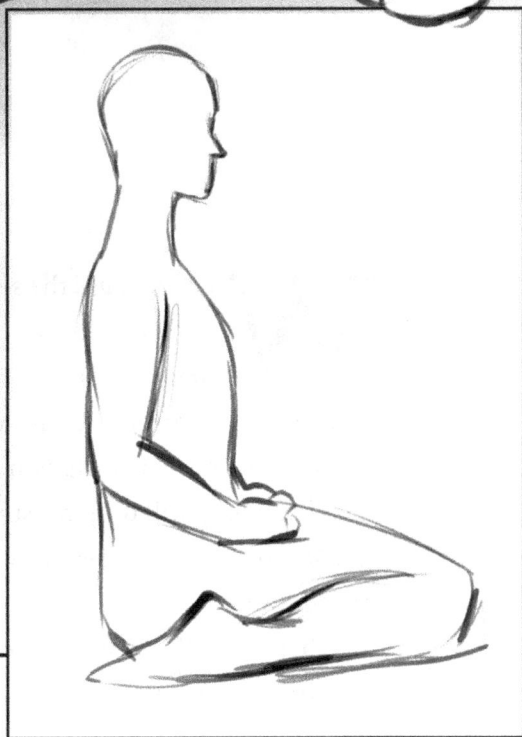

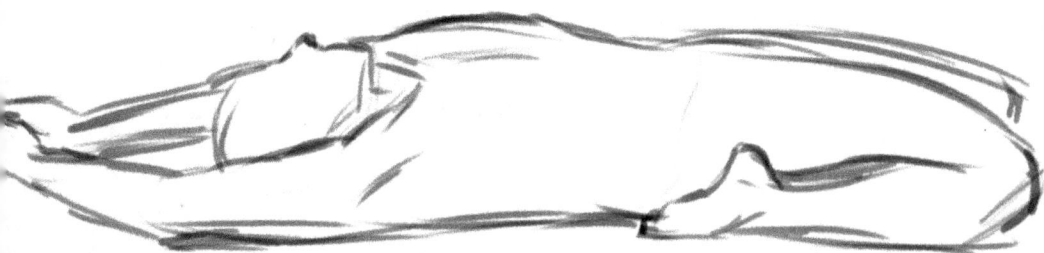

11

Diving Into Adventure in Search of Deep Knowledge

When you use the systems view as a lens to understand human activity, a field of knowledge, or any critical topic in society or life, it is essential to be aware of a principle from the theorist who pioneered this approach, the Austrian biologist Ludwig von Bertalanffy. Let's take it slow, and then the penny will drop for sure.

As you might know, a system is a set of integrated parts in continuous dynamic motion. The parts are always working together, even if we don't perceive it. You might think you're at absolute rest when you sleep at night, but your brain and body are busy cleaning up various forms of mental, emotional, and physical toxicity that you've accumulated during the day. This occurs because the system performs specific functions to achieve its purposes. These functions characterize the system as a whole.

Some of these functions are easily recognizable and explicit, while others are more subtle and implicit.

You can understand the Kaiut Yoga method as having a primary function that is easily identifiable: increasing body mobility, which in turn promotes health and longevity. Additionally, the method has a less tangible, underlying purpose: to provide practitioners with the opportunity to expand their consciousness—both of their body and their own being—as a complex whole that encompasses life itself.

For this dynamism to occur, the principle from Bertalanffy that interests us here is the existence of catalysts. These catalysts are components of the system that function like springs, triggering the dynamic processes that give the system life. They act as the procedural axis that propels the system into motion. Imagine a magnet attracting the necessary forces for the system to function as a whole, initiating a systemic whirl. In other words, it sets everything within the system into motion, activating life itself.

Your body is not a machine, contrary to the long-held and mistaken belief propagated by society's mechanistic metaphor. Instead, it is a living network of interacting forces producing energy and motion. It resembles a pulsating dance, striving to make us increasingly whole. This dynamic process aims to realize the hidden potential within us, harmonizing our individuality with the grand and encompassing dance of Nature that envelops us.

So now you might ask, "That's fine, but... What are the catalysts in the Kaiut Yoga method?"

In the body, the joints. In the process as a whole, education. The student of the method is guided to understand this through active listening. This creates a kind of magic that leads the body to a much deeper place. It fosters a lucidity that integrates multiple levels of understanding simultaneously: the perception of movement, the body's reactions, any emotions that arise, and mental awareness, all comes together.

My path of discovery was through physical pain, the horrible pain in my knees, legs, and back. It was also through the pain of losing Malu. And at various times the pain related to the story of defamation in my first marriage. And it opened up when acceptance came into my life—and acceptance that carried a deeply spiritual aura, something that felt much bigger than me, you know? When there was this deep acceptance of what seemed impossible to solve, there appeared to be room for a solution.

From there, I thought, wow, if there is a path to healing within a yoga position, this path needs to encompass everything. I began to experiment, within one of the most basic positions. I started trying to figure out how to rescue my knees in a therapeutic process. This position involves kneeling on the floor and sitting between your feet. It has a name in Sanskrit, but Americans aptly call it the Child's Pose.

It was a pleasing success for my knees because it embodied the essence of a child at play—kneeling on the floor, on the grass, with the natural ease and mobility inherent to a child's body. Initially, I believed that this mobility was the core of the rescue the position proposed.

I sought to understand where the position was born. At first glance, it appeared to be simply a kneeling posture, sitting on the floor. However, with deeper analysis, I realized that the position actually begins with the toes. I then realized that the essential rescue was *more profound. It was about restoring the biomechanical mobility of the toes.*

That's when I began the process of unblocking, both energetically and structurally, starting with my feet, then my ankles, and finally my knees. I used a position that initially seemed impossible and unfeasible for me, given that my knees were literally rotten. That's why on weekends I often chose to stay in the dark, seeking a place of rescue through simple things like images, dreams, and experimental movements I performed in bed.

Self-perception, observing my students, and comprehending Ravi's hip condition all contributed to a developing map of understanding. This map connected different times and diverse motives, forming an integrated knowledge that would eventually flow into the method.

Given my story, including being shot in the hip, I eventually realized that the root of my spinal issues, leg problems, and stiffness was actually in the hip. We often associate pain with the problem's location, but pain does not necessarily occur at the source of the imbalance.

Countless times, I observed that issues in my students' thoracic spines were biomechanically the cause of their chronic shoulder and neck problems. Many of these students underwent shoulder surgeries that only addressed the symptoms, not the root cause. Therefore, it's crucial to differentiate between pain, the problem, and the primary cause.

In my case, the primary cause was hip trauma from the firearm accident. The pain manifested in my sacroiliac region, lower back, neck, and legs, pains very far from the primary cause. There was also the phenomenon of trauma, an episode that was emotionally blocked from my conscious memory, making it difficult to connect the dots. I gradually moved from the periphery toward the hip, until I realized: "Oh, gee, the hip, the gunshot". This led to a conscious recollection of the memory and a better understanding of what had happened.

It took a long time, but this journey deepened my understanding of natural health, emphasizing that pain should not be confused with your reason for being or existing. Except for trauma caused by an accident, the source of pain often lies hidden elsewhere, typically in places that don't hurt due to compensatory processes.

Why?

The brain works on demand. For Ed, the writer working on this book, it's crucial to be one hundred percent comfortable in his chair, sitting in front of the computer and writing. He tells his brain that this is his number one priority. Once the task is finished, he reflects and asks himself, "What do I want now?" The answer might be, " I want to see my girlfriend."

What does the brain do next?

Neuroplastically, it tries to give everything it can, continually finding compensatory routes to overcome problems and deliver what you want at that moment. Does that make sense to you?

When pain appears, it's often a compensation of a compensation of a compensation. It's like a soccer ball repeatedly hitting the goalpost; no matter how many attempts are made, the shot can no longer find its way into the goal. At this point, the brain can no longer compensate, and you no longer associate the pain with its original cause.

How could I associate the pain and chronic stiffness in my neck with a gunshot wound in the hip? I worked on my neck, shoulder, back—everything, but nothing provided sustainable relief. For a long time, I couldn't see the connection between these issues. It wasn't until

I discovered the root blockage in my hip that I was able to produce a systemic impact far greater than anything I had achieved before.

From this realization came an intimacy with the hip, leading to the development of techniques and procedures focused on hip positions. I understood that today's sedentary society suffers from underutilized and weakened hips, it's a bit like a collective, societal trauma. From a natural and biomechanical standpoint, the pelvis serves as a central axis, influencing the entire body's structure and movement. By addressing the pelvis, we can generate a positive impact on the whole body.

Later, I also saw this play out in Ravi because of his hip disease. One day, he asked me:

"Dad, why don't I have pain anymore?"

"You don't have pain anymore because I broke a sweat to develop a lot of techniques to prevent the pain from settling in."

Developing the method and its application was an increasingly refined process. Many people started coming to me with chronic hip pain, femoral head arthrosis, and medical indications for hip prosthesis. I observed that many lumbar spine discomforts also originated from the hip. I delved into the issues of the hip joints, the pelvis as a whole, lower back pain, and knee problems. By seeing how these elements are interconnected, I discovered increasingly efficient therapeutic routes.

From there, I created the theory of the three girdles. The concept of the pelvic girdle—comprising the hip bones, sacrum, and lower limbs—was already known. Similarly, the shoulder girdle, which includes the clavicle and scapula, connects the chest to the upper limbs. However, I realized that a crucial part was missing.

I began to theorize the idea of a third girdle, the plantar girdle, encompassing the ankles and feet. I realized that there is an intimate biomechanical relationship between these three girdles. These are the three primary areas of impact, and anything that happens in them reverberates quickly and precisely throughout the rest of the body.

Science in action. Root science. This is the essence of this chapter in our story—the story of developing the method and its conceptual foundations. It's a tale of adventure and discovery, navigating the uncertain and dark path of the beginning without knowing if light will eventually shine. Empirical science in its original sense. Applied science is born from experimentation, observation, and testing on oneself and others, gradually uncovering the functional processes of what you research.

In this specific context, with a keen eye on the phenomenon, Francisco even prefers to replace the word "consciousness" with "lucidity." Whether we call it consciousness or lucidity, the pursuit of its expansion lies at the heart of all meaningful knowledge and practical application. However, true expansion requires meeting the challenge of integration—bringing together the broader vision with the intricate details. This integration means harmonizing the tangible, material aspects of reality with the subtle, often unseen forces that drive the dynamic movement sustaining life—whether at the scale of galaxies or within the intricacies of the human body.

The compensations that occur are not separate, dissociated problems. Everything is part of the same problem. You fall off a horse in childhood, sustaining a significant hip injury. You're a child, you may not even remember it. You're flexible and very healthy at the cellular level, but the trauma impacts that joint and molds the cartilage in a certain way. However, your priority is to be a happy and active child, so the brain tries to provide that for you. Instead of dealing with the discomfort directly, it generates compensations.

One day, you'll be an adult. That hip may become stiff, and discomfort might arise in a seemingly unrelated area, like the shoulder. However, it's not that the discomfort originates in the shoulder. It's the same hip discomfort that has generated biomechanical consequences and traveled through the body, altering tissues, lines of force, and structures. The outcome of this compensation process varies based on the individual's history, their mental processes, emotional system, how their body has been used over time, stress patterns, and other factors.

Compensations occur mainly through the relationship between the labyrinthine system involved in our balance and gravity. Gravity acts on the body from top to bottom, creating gravitational lines of force, while the body reacts to gravity from the bottom up. This interaction can lead to distortions in our response to gravity. A response wherein the brain seeks to address a fundamental priority that you've set for it.

When you wake up in the morning and get out of bed, your absolute priority is to stand up. The brain does everything possible to achieve this without pain. When pain becomes unavoidable, it means you've reached the limit of possible compensations.

The method's work in the classroom involves taking a trip back in time, reopening compensatory routes that have become overloaded and closed. That's why my goal isn't just for you to improve. I want you to regain the mobility and neuroplasticity you had at 20. This can only be achieved by moving correctly—not aggressively—through pain and limitations, thereby rescuing and cleansing your system of the stories and compensations that live in you.

There's always an emotional component to this story. Everything that remains in the body for a while becomes entangled with emotions. Suppose you had an accident and broke one of your ankles. Within a few months, this injury becomes linked with your emotional system, whether you consciously realize it or not.

The method offers a form of rescue because every trauma involves an internal split, leading to a reduction in the ability to perceive. By rewiring the system, you enhance your ability to perceive yourself in structural, bodily, and more subtle ways. You start to recover the ability to sense the body's relationship with the subtle.

For me, the separation between mind and body does not exist. It is an illusion created by our need to compartmentalize everything. However, it is the body that thinks, and it is the mind that encompasses the body, making them inseparable. And the emotional system is an integral part of this unity.

What have I noticed over the years with these rescues?

I've seen people become more capable of perceiving subtleties about themselves. From an early age, I understood the importance of complementary therapeutic processes outside the classroom for achieving a good therapeutic outcome in the classroom. Well-trained students tend to better understand the logic and process of Kaiut Yoga.

When I notice that a student responds better than average to the method, I suggest they follow up with psychotherapy from a trusted professional. Transforming the body also transforms the entire mental, emotional, and energetic model implanted in the body. When you begin to dismantle this psychic aggregate—because the body is a product of the mind—the mind has the opportunity to recognize itself. If, at this moment, the student has reliable professional therapeutic support, the process is much healthier and more complete.

From an early age, I understood that introducing psychotherapeutic content in a clinical sense into the method would be a mistake. In the yoga universe, this often leads to an intellectualization of the process, resulting in superficiality rather than genuine understanding. The individual begins to experience sensations but stays trapped within their personal history, models, and assumptions with which they have been influenced.

What I saw a lot in the yoga world was that people who practiced for a long time still had overactive minds, were as anxious as everyone else, had low resilience to stress, did not achieve calmness, aged, and sometimes got sicker than those who did not do yoga. I understood that yoga did better for those who practiced little. However, for those who practiced extensively, it appeared to generate some mental strain, burning out a few threads.

I realized that there was an error in the process. The mistake lay precisely in incorporating half-psychotherapeutic jargon into the classroom and discussing the relationship between mind and body.

I couldn't allow this contamination. The method needed to offer a process of education. It had to be profound but couldn't use any of the conventional language of yoga because that language was flawed.

Francisco's confidence in the method's development and its effective delivery of results steadily solidified over time. This assurance grew from his own personal experience, Ravi's case, and the promising outcomes of the students he taught in his first laboratory. Among these early successes was Albino Tramontina, whose story you encountered in the previous chapter. Another notable case soon followed—that of Carlos Beltrão.

Carlos:

I am 64 years old and began practicing yoga in June 1999 in one of Francisco's first classes. I am retired from the City of Curitiba but continue to work as an independent consultant in the environmental sector. I practice yoga by either following the method's online classes at home or attending an in-person class once a week at Norberto Sampaio's school, an accredited teacher located about 600 meters [a third of a mile] from my home at the Parque São Lourenço neighborhood. I am in good physical condition, training footvolley three times a week, and I have even reached the finals of the Brazilian championship for seniors over 40 years old. I have always influenced many people to practice yoga, including my wife, sister-in-law, sister, son, friends, and many others.

I was a successful indoor soccer athlete, starting when I was 17 years old. I played for prominent clubs in the states of Paraná and Santa Catarina and was even drafted for the Brazilian National Team, winning individual awards as well. However, this sport is very impactful and aggressive. I ended my career, but in 1992, I accepted invitations to play field soccer and did very well, playing in various locations. However, I began experiencing increasing problems with my ankles and knees, making it difficult to continue playing.

Albino Tramontina recommended Francisco to me. I spent two years doing chiropractic treatment with him before he started teaching yoga classes. During our first session in 1997, I mentioned my ankle problem, but he saw that my hip was crooked. He asked if I had ever had a muscle injury in my left leg. I had indeed suffered such an injury in 1992. I had gone to kick a ball, but a player from the opposing team, who was on the Brazilian National Team, intercepted me, causing my leg to open wide. I was unable to play for 20 days. The hip had dislocated to compensate for the muscle that had become shortened.

Five years later, Francisco said to me that he could fix it but that we would need to work hard, adding that if the hip returned to its place within 15 days, it would mean the body had reacted well. In fact, the muscles did react, and the

186

hip returned to its place. From there, I realized I had many more old problems to address. I had jaw surgery, and I'm not sure if it was done poorly or if it was simply very aggressive. A lot of issues in my body also stemmed from car and motorcycle accidents.

But I moved on with life and improved through the practice of yoga. The method's results were swift in many aspects. Although I still feel pain in my ankles when walking on the sidewalk, it doesn't stop me from playing footvolley, which is now my sport. I train with guys in their early 20s, and my breathing capacity is impressive. They often ask me if I get tired after an hour of training, but I continue to train well. Some aspects or my health may never be one hundred percent, but overall, everything is very satisfactory and functional. During my annual medical check-ups, I consistently achieve excellent results. In other words, I win medals.

When I started yoga, the method was not yet fully developed. Francisco was in the early stages of creating it. Initially, we practiced postures that are no longer part of the method. In a way, we were guinea pigs, but we trusted that the results would come over time. I knew it was important to provide feedback to Francisco, although many failed to do so, which was a missed opportunity. I formed a small group that went out for coffee after classes on Monday, Wednesday, and Friday before heading to work. We discussed the class, and I encouraged those with issues to speak to Francisco. Not everyone did. Some people had pain so deeply ingrained that when medication no longer worked, they gave up on the class.

I spoke up. Once, I told Francisco that a movement in class had affected my knee. He adjusted it right away. Over time, I believe he refined the method to become increasingly therapeutic, ensuring that no mistakes occurred in the classes. He continues to develop this method to this day.

Perhaps Carlos is right, in a sense. The method is solid, consistent, and coherent, but it is also in continuous development and improvement. Life is a movement from the seemingly imperfect towards the perfect reality that awaits our expanded capacity to perceive it. All the time.

When we respond to the call of this progressive adventure of discovery, we begin to understand the magnificent systemic process that is life, embodied in you and in me. We are (re)discovering elements of this process that lead us from pain to lucidity, though we may not fully understand it yet.

Fascia is a connective tissue that loses flexibility and adheres after trauma, injury, or chronic tension. It is integral in the very literal sense of the word. Therefore, you have nothing to do with fascia but to return it to its normal state, which ensures an ideal and youthful tone. Fascia is designed to maintain this state as long as the body remains fluid in its natural design.

When you lose movement, it creates a snowball effect. The loss of movement leads to a decrease in the vitality of the fascia, which in turn causes issues in various other tissue relationships. This process begins to move in opposition to the natural crank of life. What people often refer to as aging involves a series of losses, and while there may be some truth to that, I believe that aging primarily results from the lack of correct movement. The lack of balance in the harmonic movement of the whole body.

The method offers a process to restore the vitality a person could naturally have today if they had kept proper care. It is a return to the normal state of nature. I want new cells to regenerate under the positive influence of beneficial stimuli. The key to this process is joint work, which is crucial in unlocking and recovering the functional fascia. Contrary to what many believe, fascia is not an active agent in this process. It is passive and simply responds to stimuli. However, it is essential to provide the right stimuli.

I want to rescue functions with high neural connectivity so that the rescue sets the mechanism of Nature itself in motion. Because Nature is adaptable. She heals herself.

You go to Praça da Sé, the central square in the old and polluted center of São Paulo, where there are many beggars and stray dogs. Despite these harsh conditions, you find a patch of grass struggling to thrive. Even in the toughest environments, Nature strives to prosper. It takes a significant counterforce to prevent it from flourishing.

It's the same logic. From working with the first people who came to me with knee, shoulder, and hip problems, I learned that if you provide a minimal, natural functional stimulus, Nature will regenerate. This minimum is the basic logic of the method. It has nothing to do with aesthetics, it has nothing to do with muscles.

As you read this, did you begin to imagine that the method increasingly resonates with the idea that Nature heals itself? Did it cross your mind Nature's intrinsic wisdom leads to health and well-being?

These questions also grew in Francisco's mind. To seek answers and added assurance, Francisco embarked on a voyage of exploration... to Tibet!

I took a sabbatical. I went to Tibet because I wanted to see a population less influenced by the distorted modern logic of comfort and avoidance of sensation, which actually kills more than anything else. Through my work with students, I had already understood that the path to recovering function passes through pain, not analgesia. Analgesia preserves the problem, not the person.

Analgesia can even be natural. You can use acupuncture to alleviate pain. You can get a massage, go to therapy, or take a painkiller. All these falls into the category of avoiding pain.

But the rescue goes through pain in the right way, with the correct dose and time. The process requires the proper explanation, too. You must nurture the intellect so the individual can withstand the emotions during the therapeutic process. There cannot be a therapeutic process of this magnitude without the individual understanding the process, understanding the whys, and dealing with their pain head-on in a very adult, mature way, without any aggressiveness. It asks for individuals to enter a unique place internally, where the process dismantles false premises and creates a systemic therapeutic domino effect.

What I saw in Tibet shocked me. Of course, the influence of the modern world is everywhere now, and no place is completely shielded from it. Even so, I saw people over 90 squatting on the floor or kneeling, getting up and down, and displaying a childlike, natural mobility in the truest sense of the word. I saw very elderly adults in the nomadic population with a level of physical capacity and adaptability. This brought me further certainty concerning the method.

The definitive certainty was that the Kaiut Yoga method was naturally aligning with the wisdom of life manifested on this beautiful blue planet. This realization set the stage for the method's expansion—through teacher training courses and an unexpected yet organic international growth, with the United States at its core.

However, as with all journeys in life, this path is marked by challenges, progress, and occasional setbacks. To move in harmony with the natural rhythm of evolution and expansion, one must embrace the reality that growth is an ongoing process—requiring us to continuously learn new steps in the intricate, systemic dance of existence. It has always been this way, and it always will be. There is no other way forward but to dive in—wholeheartedly, with heart, mind, and soul.

12

Of Coincidences That Do Not Exist and Other Mysteries That Do

The beginning of Francisco's journey along the path of teacher training was frankly frustrating and unpromising. As the classic poem by celebrated Brazilian poet Carlos Drummond de Andrade says, "in the middle of the road there was a stone, there was a stone in the middle of the road."

Riding on the poetic gaze helps us realize how much hidden poetry is intertwined with life and its real stories. It opens our perspective to the unusual angles that poets often see, angles we might overlook due to the prevailing societal discourse that simplifies existence. The danger lies in getting caught up in this reductionism, which can numb us to the complex richness of the universe that weaves together the fate of people and stories of transformative innovation like this one. It's important to note that, within the narrative, there may be more than one obstacle.

Sometimes, rather than a literal stone, these challenges can be abstract, subtle, yet equally uncomfortable.

I was very resistant to the idea of training teachers. Even when I started, I was super skeptical. I didn't feel any certainty that I should be doing it. I didn't feel ready, nor inclined. I didn't even think the method was fully developed. I questioned whether the informal environment of a yoga room was suitable for teaching theoretical content. Although I had good lesson plans, my chronic discomfort stemmed from not having the method's logic well established. I suspected that delivering better teachers to the market would be a significant challenge.

What were the challenges?

The first challenge was the market's low expectations of yoga. It is typically seen as merely a physical practice focused on body positions and performance. This shallow perception downgraded the discipline's potential impact. The general public, in turn, say yoga in a negative light, further complicating its acceptance. Another significant challenge was my own lack of awareness about what was truly needed to elevate and teach yoga effectively.

People, however, began to recognize my work, and soon people came from other states to Curitiba, eager to train with me or work at the school. I realized there was a pent-up demand and an untapped opportunity that I could fulfil.

The average understanding of most who came to me in the beginning could have been higher. They were stuck in an old pattern. Historically, during its classical development, yoga was revolutionary. However, from the 1940s onward, as yoga spread worldwide, it became superficial. It turned into just another tool in the repertoire of teachers in physical education and the physical therapies. Yoga had been stripped of its cutting-edge characteristics.

I saw, however, that many teachers were ethical individuals who had a genuine desire to do good for others. This motivated me, along with the fact that I had accumulated a substantial amount of information by then. I had studied the works of great visionaries of human development, including Rudolf Steiner, and incorporated my chiropractic knowledge. Combining all of this, I developed my own way of teaching yoga.

Even before the logic of the method was fully developed, I was already presenting it as the spontaneous, half-intuitive approach that it is. Pure poetry!

When students arrived for the first teacher training course, I knew the method wasn't fully developed. Nevertheless, they were met with an immense theoretical load, packed with technical complexity, which disrupted the market's usual lack of content. There was a noticeable gap between the method and the students' lack of understanding of what constitutes quality yoga practice. I also observed that many had fragile bodies and lacked the physical structure needed for the practice they aimed to undertake. They were not prepared to face the pain.

It is charming to appreciate someone wonderfully playing the guitar, with the chords naturally flowing in melody. However, delivering genuine quality takes thousands of hours of practice, exercise, and repetition. This was the big shock I had with my students. They didn't understand this. They wanted to mimic the practice, copying ideas and words as if it were a mere performance. They were convinced that the method was just a set of excellent class plans, not realizing that the plans were merely tools within the broader method.

Everyone came to the course wanting more, seemingly eager to learn, but in reality, many didn't study, dedicate themselves, or practice. They were upset when they received content that was not a cake recipe, some step-by-step process. Some people have this habit. They don't strive to be great. They want the minimum.

It seems my figure was romanticized there. But in reality, I was a super technical guy. I simply wanted to deliver good content and ensure great teachers emerged from the program. I never had any other motives.

Ah, the eternal obstacle of innovators; the universal dilemma of revolutionaries who bring new knowledge to the world; the greatest challenge for those who rejuvenate society: being misunderstood or ignored. Human nature tends to view today's transformative innovations through the blurred lenses of yesterday, and in doing so, people miss the point.

I didn't understand why some of these students left. I had no conflict with them, but they began to curse me. On their part, an actual conflict arose, perhaps a conflict of possession or jealousy over the content, the number of students I had, the profound simplicity and efficiency of the techniques I developed, and the results they delivered. Many of them went on to promote themselves, claiming they understood my work better than I did and that they had better versions to offer.

There were some situations where I was ticked off. But externally, I never reacted. It's like the story of the rejected scientist. What does he do? He goes back to the lab and starts the experiment again. Someone with real consistency and love for what they do stays focused and gets back to work, even when someone speaks ill of them. But someone without a life, soul, or passion for their work has time to speak ill of others. A person who spends mental energy cursing others is already sick, fragile, and lacks consistency. In not reacting, the verbal attacks would simply pass and disappear with time. My approach of not saying anything or reacting turned out to be very efficient.

For the first teacher training course, Francisco organized around twelve topics and worked on them intensively, meeting one weekend per month for a year. Although he initially felt incredible frustration with the results, this discomfort didn't paralyze him for long. Instead, it motivated him to improve those around him and himself. This process became a journey of maturation as a teacher, the evolution of his method, and even the growth of the public seeking him out. He established a habit of continuous improvement in the courses, enhancing language, communication processes, and didactic aspects.

Lúcia Torres was a student in the first class in 2009. Over time, she would become the longest-serving teacher, working at Francisco's school in Curitiba. At the time of writing, she continues to work at the Batel school, now under Ravi's leadership. Her connection to the Kaiut clan dates back even further and has taken various forms over the years.

I was 34 years old when I separated. I moved from Paranaguá—a nearby port city—to Curitiba with my three children to rebuild my life. It was a traumatic experience, including for my parents, especially my father, who developed an ulcer that the family came to refer to as "Lucia's Ulcer." My children were deeply affected as well; they had to leave behind a big house, a housekeeper, and all the comforts they were used to.

In addition to the emotional trauma, I suffered from severe lower back pain that had worsened over the years, especially during my pregnancies. I began getting weekly massages from Antonio, and sometimes from Francisco when his father was traveling. After ten years of massages, Francisco sat next to me one day and asked,

"How much longer are you going to come to relieve back pain without wondering why you have this pain?"

His question prompted me to start practicing yoga with him, while continuing my massages with Antonio.

Lúcia had four years away from the Kaiuts, during which time she pursued yoga elsewhere; managed a clothing business with her sister, which eventually had to close; and navigated family dramas, including a son's severe illness requiring a bone marrow transplant, and the death of another son. After all that, Lúcia accepted an invitation to work at the new school Francisco had opened in Praça da Espanha.

She was hired as a classroom assistant. The school was booming, with about 200 students by her estimate. She was surprised by the profile of the students, which included many people who had never done yoga before and a sizable number of more mature students. The school offered eight classes per day. Besides Francisco and Luciana, another teacher also led classes.

In her role, Lúcia attended many of Francisco's classes, prepared the room for activities, and learned how he utilized the wall and the floor. When the third teacher resigned, Lucia had to take over those classes. Taking her first teacher training course in 2009 was a natural step in her path to qualification. She closely tracked the development of the method and Francisco's evolution as a teacher.

The method was in development since 2001. When they opened the Batel school in Praça da Espanha, Francisco had the freedom to implement his beliefs fully. Initially, he was very authoritarian, enforcing his ideas without much explanation. If you didn't understand, you should leave, you know? However, he has since evolved into a wise teacher who explains what is happening and helps others understand.

Today, he has a natural ability to observe a student, to look at someone who is working with him, and see what is not working properly. And he approaches the person and shares what he sees.

He has also been a mentor to me, my lifelong teacher, not just in yoga—I am incredibly grateful to him. Like Antonio, who inspires people and helped me during a tough time when my son was in the hospital, Francisco has taught me a lot about strength. Not that I felt like a victim, but anyway...

She recollects sharing a challenging experience with Francisco, whose response was, let's say, provocative.

He then asked... "so, did you run to your brother, your mother, and your father? You will never grow up like this, damn it!"

And then, with a witty smile, she makes me understand that Francisco has changed. She doesn't say it outright, but the relief in her expression speaks volumes... let's move on...

From the second edition of the teacher training course onwards, which was didactically perfected by Francisco's self-criticism, the profile of those who sought him out changed substantially for the better. It began attracting people who recognized themselves as receptive to his approach, some of whom had no prior experience with any form of yoga. Many were drawn by personal suffering from their experiences of pain and felt a calling to qualify as teachers, aiming to bring others the educational-therapeutic benefits they had experienced themselves through the evolving method. The gradual growth of this community multiplied the method's reach and provided a new way of working in the future, with the accreditation of exclusive schools founded by teacher-entrepreneurs under the Kaiut Yoga label.

One of these pioneers was the general practitioner and pediatrician, Norberto Sampaio.

I learned about the method in 2010, about a year after surgery for a herniated disc. My wife, Maria Leny, who had also undergone spinal surgery, and I attended an experimental class at the Praça da Espanha school. The teacher was Lúcia Torres.

I soon understood the logic of moving your body to recover function. I began practicing twice a week. In parallel, I continued weight training, running on weekends, and swimming long distances—three thousand meters [just under two miles], three times a week. I continued those activities for a year, until I tore the rotator cuff in my right shoulder. I had to undergo surgery.

I stopped all other activities completely and focused solely on yoga. I managed to keep muscle function and structure while gaining flexibility. When Francisco opened a new teacher training course the following year, I enrolled. However, I couldn't complete the course in 2013 because I couldn't fulfill the mandatory internship due to my job as a civil servant at the Federal Revenue Service in Curitiba. By then, I had moved away from Medicine. I retired in 2014 and joined the next class to complete the internship and finish my training.

From then on, I dedicated myself exclusively to yoga, spending the next few years completing over a thousand hours of internship. Francisco often remarked that I was practically living at the school in Praça da Espanha. I accompanied him in the classroom, spent a lot of time with the teachers, and observed the students.

It was a privilege to witness Francisco's ability to see each person and understand the impact of body misuse on various systems, such as the digestive system and hips. He could perceive patterns of restrictions based on an individual's personal history, gender, age, and ethnic background. He shares this expertise with those who are deeply connected and willing to learn.

My goal was to return to the health field with a different perspective from what I had as a doctor, combining my medical knowledge with this effective yoga method. I intended to open my own school. While building it, I completed an internship at the main school—which was such a privilege. I signed the licensing contract in 2015, and in March 2018, I opened the school here in Parque São Lourenço, close to home. Francisco himself gave the inaugural class.

My wife, a business administrator and retired federal employee from the Ministry of Health, and my sister Elisabete, a retired civil engineer from the municipal public service of Curitiba, are both involved in this enterprise with me. Both completed teacher training as well and now teach here with me.

We have 86-year-old students who continue to practice. We also have two seven-year-old boys who come with their mothers to practice, as well as a 13-year-old student. Remarkably, we had a student who joined at the age of 93. This is the man who married my mother-in-law after being widowed. He practiced with us for about two years, only pausing due to the COVID pandemic, some time ago.

All have achieved results. The method provides this. I have seen it happen to everyone after a sequence of classes. There are emotional improvements, reduced stress, and even better sleep for the children. There are overall improvements in the quality of life.

Even the architect who designed the project to install our school in containers, which required an electric floor heating system, became the school's number one student. She arrived here after having two spinal surgeries and no longer experiences severe pain. While she still needs to take certain precautions, she no longer faces new surgeries or major impediments in her life. She continues to work on construction sites, conducts inspections, climbs where needed, and leads an almost everyday life.

And what about me, you may ask?

When I started yoga, Francisco pointed out that I had a lot of rigidity throughout my body. In swimming, I always breathed on the right side because I couldn't turn my neck to the left. This limitation contributed to a hernia on the left side, and I had already compromised my left leg. Although it did not atrophy, it was heading in that direction. I was experiencing neurological alterations and loss of sensitivity, which led to lumbar surgery. Following that, I underwent two shoulder surgeries.

Do I still have pain?

Sporadically, yes, in the hip and lumbar areas. But it's not intense. I haven't needed to take medication again. Yoga provided relief and helped me regain functioning. Here at the school, I climb the roof, clean, do maintenance, prune trees, and handle everything necessary. If I overexert myself, I might experience some consequences, but as soon as I practice yoga, it alleviates any remaining pain and restores my mobility.

How do I see Francisco and the method today?

I see a professional dedicated to expanding the method he developed to reach as many people as possible. He practices what he preaches and applies it with the necessary care to his students. It is a replicable method. I have accompanied Francisco in training hundreds of teachers. The logic behind the method, which can be adopted by schools, is proving to be a success everywhere.

Norberto's comments on the present and leap into the future, calls us to step back into the past to clearly visualize the full story. There was no immediate rise to glory, nor maturation without stumbling blocks.

To understand this properly, it is worth remembering that coincidences do not exist. Instead, meaningful and seemingly mysterious synchronies do. These unseen cosmic forces, much like subterranean rivers, shape and influence the visible streams of our lives, subtly guiding us toward deeper understanding. In doing so, they illuminate a grander, more profound narrative—one rich with potential and meaning, waiting to be discovered.

But without action, nothing manifests. The creation—born from the intricate web of mysterious synchronies as a mere possibility—will remain confined to the realm of dreams, never crossing into reality. Left untouched, its unique essence will be lost to eternity, never to arise in the same way again. This echoes the popular wisdom, that "a saint at home rarely works miracles." To be recognized as such, one must venture afield and be discovered first in the homes of others.

One day, I received an international phone call from a woman I didn't know, and who didn't know me. She was a Brazilian named Monica Cunningham, living in the United States, who hadn't set foot in Brazil for a long time. She said she was calling from Grand Junction, Colorado, and was organizing a course that would be given by the well-known teacher Nancy Stechert. She informed me that my name was on the guest list and simply wanted to know if I had accepted the invitation, so she could confirm my presence. Neither she nor I had the slightest idea how my name ended up on that list. I never managed to find out.

I went to Grand Junction to participate in Nancy's classes as a student. Even though my English was unbelievably bad, I engaged in conversations throughout the course, participated in debates, and helped some people with pain issues, because everyone experiences pain at some point. This allowed everyone to see that I was knowledgeable about what I was doing. At the very end of the course, Nancy invited me to give a demonstration class. I was already very adept in the classroom, so this demo was a game-changer for both me and everyone who took part.

Monica immediately invited me to teach at the school she was setting up in Grand Junction. Soon after, Nancy also invited me to help her set up her school in Hotchkiss, a nearby town, as a guest teacher. She extended an invitation for me to spend a season there every few months.

Grand Junction, just under 249 miles (400 kms) from Colorado's capital and largest city, Denver. In 2023 it had a population of around 69,000 and serves as the commercial center of a region famous for producing fruits, from peaches to pears, plums to apricots, and wine. This locale would provide an entry point for Francisco to experience a more rural, country lifestyle in non-cosmopolitan America.

About an hour's drive away is Hotchkiss, a small town with around 930 inhabitants. Nestled in a valley of abundant orchards and stunning views of nature, it would prove to be an ideal oasis of peace and concentration for deepening the yoga experience. Nancy was a distinguished yoga teacher with over 30 years of experience in the Iyengar tradition, having been awarded advanced certification by B.K.S. Iyengar himself in India. She had previously founded yoga centers in Denver, Tokyo, and Singapore, and decided to settle in this quiet small town, opening Hotchkiss Yoga Tree Studio in 2006.

The first time I went there, I arrived at the door and then stopped, startled. There was a picture of me and an announcement to the public, describing me as... a Brazilian healer! A healer, mind you! Healer in the most straightforward and direct sense: someone who heals other people's illness. "Damn it! Who will show up here? What do they expect from me? Who are these people?"

The people who showed up were those in pain, people with complicated health issues, and a few yoga teachers. During my first visit, I stayed for several weeks, and as I continued to return, always staying for weeks at a time, the demand from people with this profile increased. For me, it was paradise because I knew how to handle their pain.

I had the unique opportunity to work with Americans who, for the most part, had never done yoga. People from the countryside with a more traditional American mentality, not contaminated by big city values. This experience allowed me to develop my understanding of the English language and improve my fluency. I was able to test what worked in terms of language choice for the classes. All of this helped me understand the audience and the method's reach.

Nancy then arranged for me to attend some small events in Boulder. It quickly became clear how surprising and welcoming the Americans were, showing a lot of goodwill to understand what I was delivering. There was no resistance, only openness. When you have something good to deliver, it doesn't matter if you're green, purple, yellow, or blue. It doesn't matter if you have an accent. They take the time to understand you. From the beginning, they recognized that Kaiut Yoga is what yoga has always aimed to be. They understood it is the yoga everyone needs, the yoga that should be in schools, and the yoga that people should practice in the future.

Because of the work I had already been doing in Curitiba, I arrived in the United States much more prepared. I realized that the work was even better than I had imagined, given the way I was received and how quickly the concept began to be embraced.

However, in Curitiba, during this growth phase of my work, I did not receive the same welcome from the traditional yoga community. I am still opposed by this traditional Brazilian community. They try to devalue my work, arguing that what I do is not yoga.

Being received in the United States in this way, by a society always eager to consume good things, made me realize that I could not neglect the language, the method, and the courses. It had already been happening naturally, but this experience solidified my understanding that a teacher's speech alone could regulate the student's autonomic nervous system. That's why I developed a specific cadence of speech, with pauses, intonation, and inflection in my voice. This approach minimizes discursive doubt and anchors a very palpable state of presence.

Speech alone can take a student out of an anxious, sympathetic state and bring them into a parasympathetic mode, which is the state of rest. From there, we can achieve a level of cellular nutrition. I was confirming that my voice can guide the student out of this combative state, away from contact with traumatic, often violent processes and ancestral pain, into a curative and regenerative mode. It involves engaging with the pain as a vehicle for reorganization and healing. This can happen in many ways, but the fastest and most efficient method is through the interaction between a good teacher and a student who is educated to listen. This combination fosters a very robust speed of change.

From Francisco's speech, you may already be deducing that the trip to Boulder would accelerate and expand the method's development, enhancing the entry into the United States that the initial experiences in Grand Junction and Hotchkiss represented.

After all, Boulder, just 27 miles (44 kms) northwest of Denver, with a population of around 106,000 in 2023, is not only larger but also a progressive city and a significant cultural center. It is home to a community of open-minded, liberal people involved in civic activism. Naropa University, of Buddhist origin, is one of the pioneering academic institutions in contemplary education. It integrates Eastern wisdom with contemporary science and has played a role in popularizing modern mindfulness-meditation practices. This university is an integral part of the local historical scene and has a long association with yoga.

Systemically, this background perfectly aligns with Francisco's next steps in Colorado and North America. Boulder would become a natural initial base for the expansion of his work. Remember the concept of systemic catalysts? Geographically, Boulder would serve as the catalyst for this episode in his history and the development of his method.

But for things to happen, the right conditions of time, place, and means are not enough. The involvement of people remains critical in any story and will continue to be, even in this era of technological advancements like artificial intelligence. However, they can appear in your path in unusual and surprising ways.

When Francisco arrives in Boulder for the events organized by Nancy, he is not surrounded entirely by strangers. Because of those phenomena in life that we often mistake for coincidences—there really is no such thing—Nancy decided to invite him to teach in this city where a couple of her friends lived. The way he first met the woman of this couple, Helena Bolduc, was equally surprising.

Helena:

Francisco was inviting yoga teachers from the United States to come and teach his students in Brazil. He invited Richard Freeman, a renowned Ashtanga Yoga teacher from Boulder. Richard's wife, Mary Taylor, replied that Richard was not traveling abroad to teach, but they had a Brazilian yoga teacher at their studio who might be available to go.

I sent him an email,

"Look, I have a ticket to Brazil in a month and a half. If you want, I can stop by. Where are you from?"

He replied,

"Curitiba."

"Look at that! Coincidence or not, I'm from Curitiba too! That's where I'm going!"

When I arrived, I had another surprise. Francisco's school in Praça da Espanha, the previous one in the Barcelona building, was just one block away from my parents' house.

I left Curitiba in my early 20s and started traveling abroad. First, I went to London to study dance. From there, I came to the United States to study at CalArts, the California Institute of the Arts. Afterward, I moved to Boulder to study at Naropa University, where I became a Buddhist. I ended up staying here.

I didn't know Francisco's yoga. He showed me his work, but I was invited to teach Ashtanga Yoga to his teachers. The following year, I returned to Curitiba and taught more classes. About two or three years after my first visit, I returned to teach in his new space, right there in the Square, where they had built a charming duplex. This time, I came back to teach meditation. I decided to take his yoga classes as a student, and I found the method amazing!

We became very good friends with Francisco, my husband David and I. About five years after our first visit to him in Curitiba, David joined me, and Francisco came to give his first lessons in Hotchkiss. We then invited him to stay at our house in Boulder whenever he was in the area. Eventually, his whole family came, his wife at the time, his father, and his son, Ravi. From then on, he stayed at our house every time he passed through Boulder or came to teach. This developed into an enjoyable and intimate family friendship.

For my part, I believe my relationship with Francisco is very karmic, much like my friendship with Richard Freeman. There came a point in my life when I stopped being a yoga teacher. I preferred to be friends with Francisco rather than a yoga teacher he worked with, just as I prefer to be Richard's friend rather than one of his teachers.

No longer a teacher, but always a friend, I informally supported initiatives to expand the method as a business in Boulder. David, a yoga practitioner, who at one point also became Francisco's student, used his expertise as a businessperson and spontaneous cultural promoter to help our Brazilian friend on his American journey.

The Bolduc's owns the largest and trendiest independent bookstore in the city, the Boulder Book Store. It is conveniently located in a pedestrian-only shopping center on Pearl Street, houses more than 100,000 titles across three floors, and serves as a vibrant center of cultural events. It has hosted guest authors such as Gloria Steinem, Joyce Carol Oates, Stephen King, Deepak Chopra, and Elizabeth Gilbert.

David:

I'm from Michigan, but I was living in California during the Vietnam War. I became incredibly involved in the anti-war movements and started taking part full-time. That's why I moved here to Colorado, to continue my involvement in the anti-war movement.

I opened a small bookstore in Denver in 1968. Then, around 1973, I moved to Boulder and opened our bookstore here. I came to Boulder because I wanted to study with a Buddhist teacher from Tibet and be close to the Buddhist community.

The friendship with Francisco developed gradually. Sometimes, he came with his wife and children. We have welcomed him into our home many times. On one of his recent visits, I took him to a place I have in the desert in Southern California and left him there for a week. It had been a long time since he had the opportunity to rest and relax.

Later, I went to meet him, and we flew together to San Francisco. From there, I rented a beach house further north, where we stayed for about two weeks. It was hilarious because, at night, when I wanted to watch a movie or something, he would put himself in a yoga posture and make me hold the same posture throughout the entire movie...

When Francisco started his own classes here in Boulder, we supported him. We found a place for him to rent for his classes and publicized the event on the bookstore's website, which has about 10,000 followers. Initially, we rented spaces in churches with large halls. We had a good relationship with the churches here, so as his number of students grew, we continued to rent their spaces.

Helena:

We wanted to give Francisco all the support possible. We spread the word to friends, and I personally attended his classes as a student. David also started attending at a certain point. Our network of contacts within the yoga community was extensive. Largely because for a few years, our business, was involved with the Yoga Journal Conference, run by the well-known trade magazine of the time, *Yoga Journal*. This was a nationwide program of major yoga events, including a local version in the Boulder region.

I also helped by finding someone here to organize his visits, promote events, and attract new students. He started coming every year. Everyone who attended his classes loved them, and they would return for the next session. The classrooms became more and more crowded, with many people eager to join the classes. That's how he became known in Boulder.

When a trio of Francisco's students—a woman and two men—expressed their dream of opening a yoga studio in the city, dedicated to his method, I initially helped them. I suggested potential rental spaces and assisted with the promotion to get them started.

Do I have an explanation for yet another factor that contributes to his success here in Boulder?

The yoga boom in the United States coincided with its emergence here. In Boulder, yoga was already well known because of Richard Freeman's work, which attracted people from all over the world to take classes with him. There were many yoga groups. Just 40 minutes from here, the Yoga Journal Conference took place. This conference, along with the associated newspaper—later a magazine—played a significant role in disseminating yoga in the area. Everyone in Boulder was curious about yoga. Those who had never practiced it started, and even those who did not practice were aware of it because everyone had a friend or acquaintance who did.

However, several lines of yoga are quite demanding to practice. You need a certain type of physique or be a particular age. Suddenly, Francisco arrived with a yoga method suitable for everyone. It worked out incredibly well! He arrived at the right place at the right time. That was his moment, more than any other yoga teacher's. It was his karma. It had to happen then.

Francisco comments that this expansion did not result from a structured, planned movement. It was loose and spontaneous. Even when things took off for good, the work he had set up in Curitiba became destabilized due to the dissolution of his marriage with Luciana and the parental custody issue with Malu. Additionally, there was his personal resistance to travel, because he loves his routine of waking up at half past five in the morning, practicing yoga, having coffee with his partner, teaching yoga classes, practicing yoga again, teaching another class, and doing more yoga...

I traveled reluctantly. I would leave feeling resentful, and came back feeling the same way...

He had terrible jet lag, which is understandable given that he spent his life nurturing his body with care. Suddenly, he found himself in a travel routine that disrupted his usual healthy habits.

However, he found compensation in the challenge of making himself understood in a new language, the gratifying feeling of seeing his work recognized, and the temporary relief from the heavy wear and tear he faced at home.

The work was expanding magnificently in Boulder and other parts of the United States that Francisco had never considered.

That's when a new student from Toronto, who attended some classes in Boulder, brought a new proposal to Francisco. Introducing herself as a highly competent executive in the advertising world, she convinced Francisco that to be successful internationally, it would be better to do it from Canada. And then...

I'll tell you the truth. I was very naïve.

13

Into Deep America and Beyond

I f we return to Helena's comment—that there are karmic times and places people's lives—we can perhaps think it inevitable that Francisco's journey and success would come through Colorado and the United States. Time and place working together to create the potential for destiny. As, Helena said, he was the right person in the right place at the right time.

However, even where fate and destiny are concerned, there is an element of free will. Opportunities must be seized with determination, otherwise the karmic potential—whether positive, for growth, or negative, hindering progress—can fade away. Without action, the protagonist risks losing direction, stalling personal growth, and preventing the story from fully unfolding.

Colorado is Francisco's karmic place par excellence, especially during his early days as an innovative teacher in North America.

It's not just one isolated city but the state as a whole. His work began in Grand Junction, blossomed in Hotchkiss, and now shines in Boulder as a powerful force. And it is from there that it will expand further across the region.

But what kind of energy does Colorado hold? How does it fit into the larger system of the nation it belongs to? What makes this place a gateway of opportunities for the method to be exposed to the bright light and critical examination of a new cultural landscape? What hidden meanings or implications does its name hold? What cultural, social, historical, natural, and human elements create the fertile ground for Francisco's creative act to take root?

The name "Colorado," derived from the Spanish word meaning "reddish," reflects the distinctive reddish-brown silt carried by the Colorado River that runs through the state. To look at a map of the United States, you can see that Colorado is not on the East Coast, bathed by the Atlantic, nor on the West, visited by the waters of the Pacific. Far from the oceans, it is also not at the extreme north or south of the state. It is an enclave in the mountainous west, bordering seven other states. As such, Colorado becomes a meeting point of natural contrasts: The high deserts of Utah, Arizona, and Mexico to the south and west, and the plain and prairies of Wyoming, Nebraska, Oklahoma, and Kansas to the north and east. Running straight through the state, and Boulder, is the Rocky Mountains, the long north-south route of 2990 miles (4,800 kms) descending from Canada through to New Mexico.

Beyond its geography, Colorado's history tells the story of a cultural mosaic. The Ute, Comanche, Arapaho, and Cheyenne peoples lived here long before the arrival of Spanish conquistadores and Mexican settlers. The Treaty of Guadalupe Hidalgo in 1848 transferred the territory from Mexico to the United States, ushering in waves of European, Asian, and North American immigrants drawn by the gold, silver, and copper rushes of the nineteenth and early twentieth centuries. Later, as mining waned, the region reinvented itself with tourism—epitomized by ski resorts like Aspen and Vail, and adventure tourism in its stunning parks, rivers, and mountains. In this context of leisure, wellness, and breathtaking scenery, the state became a hub for outdoor yoga festivals and retreats.

Deep America welcomed Francisco. But is this more of a "Francisco Conquers America" episode? Or the reverse? Or a hybrid phenomenon?

Let's continue on this journey together, and then, you can decide.

I had another massive surprise when dealing with this new culture of Colorado. The first was the receptivity to my work. There was not an absolute and quick acceptance, of course. But there was an acceptance far superior to anything I had ever experienced in Curitiba. When the classes began to grow and I started teaching dozens of people in church halls in Boulder, the second surprise happened.

Yoga teachers began bringing their students to my classes so they could have a direct experience with me. I was being recognized as a teacher of teachers. The Americans saw value in my work and recognized the success behind the full classrooms. They wanted to be part of it. Many of those who initially attended my classes continued to come back. They attended my classes during my following visits to the area, months later, and beyond. It was an incredible energy.

After a long time, during the later stages of my travels, major events started to occur. These events drew hundreds of people and took place in diverse settings—at the Buddhist-inspired Naropa University, within a Jewish center, and in gymnasiums featuring impressive setups. It began to feel like something out of a movie, you know?

In Boulder, especially, from the very beginning there was an interesting demand for regular classes. When I was there in-person, there were who would take classes every day, and there were people who took two to three classes daily. In some cases, people even changed professions to become yoga teachers, of my yoga. And then there were some who were traditional yoga teachers seeking a change in orientation in their career.

These seasons in the United States were never a place to make or save money. Especially because each trip like this is obviously expensive. But I saw everything as an incredibly unique opportunity, an extraordinarily rich experience. And not just for me.

Sometimes, I did everything I could so Ravi could come with me. There was a time when Ravi was with me in Boulder both times in the year I went to teach. When his school holidays in Brazil coincided with summer holidays, he spent them in Colorado. For him, who studied at a bilingual Swiss school, it was then quite easy communicate in English. He would make friends with a lot of people, with some of those friendships continuing to this day. Ravi had very enjoyable Colorado experiences.

Despite my demanding teaching schedule, I made a point to immerse myself in the cultural universe of Boulder. Even when I traveled solo, I never felt alone. I relished exploring the city's diverse locales, going to the cinema, and occasionally attending the theater.

I delved deeply into Boulder's gastronomic offerings, a pursuit that borders on a cherished hobby for me. I revel in the serendipity of *discovering restaurants spontaneously. I enjoy wandering the streets and being drawn into a place on a whim. The thrill of being surprised by the menu, exploring the wine list, and deciphering the character and essence of each locale—the "nature of the place"—is a uniquely gratifying experience.*

The nature of Boulder's culinary scene really aligns with my tastes. It strikes a balance between a strong emphasis on healthy dining and organic, local produce and a dedication to the refined artistry of haute cuisine.

The city also played a key role as an inspiring stimulus for the scholar and researcher in me. Scientists from different fields took classes with me, as well as yoga teachers of different styles. I had enriching conversations with remarkable people. I had the opportunity to see and analyze diverse patterns of body use.

Everything was profoundly enriching, especially because the unexpected often surfaced during my classes, presenting new challenges. The unpredictability of each session invigorated me, as I never knew what to expect. This dynamic aspect greatly appealed to me and eventually became a cornerstone of my future teacher training courses: the importance of being always prepared for the unexpected.

A well-known yoga teacher from Boulder, who had attended my lectures and taken some classes with me, approached me with a request. She respected my work and wanted to bring a student to see if I could assist him. She provided little detail, simply mentioning that she was finding it challenging to collaborate with him. I assumed he would be a regular practitioner facing some standard difficulties.

She was very honest and very authentic in her attitude. True to her word, she brought a young man who had suffered a brain injury from an accident. As a result, he faced significant difficulties with locomotion, experienced spasms, and had some cognitive impairments. I responded well, drawing on my ability to perceive the other person, to be fully present and attuned to each situation. I consolidated the understanding of how important it is not to be caught on the wrong foot by anything surprising that occurs in the classroom. I was elated to help both the young man and the teacher. And I learned a profound lesson: the most essential requirement is to see beyond the label and discover the person behind it.

Francisco´s role in guiding people to realize new potential, whatever their starting circumstance, wasn´t confined to Boulder. While the first teacher training course in the United States did indeed take place in Colorado, it was held in Hotchkiss, 250 miles (400 kms) away.

Among the participants were several people from Boulder. A moment of surprise came when a group of students from this class planted an idea I had not previously considered,

"This is very unique—it needs to have a name. It's original, one hundred percent original. That's why it needs to have your name!"

From there the brand was born. The name of this brand and method that until then had no name: Kaiut Yoga.

This experience was yet another shock for me. The students in Colorado took immense pride in my work and in their participation. They felt an ethical obligation to give me credit, which had a profound impact on me.

As I spoke to previously, in Brazil I often met people who expressed interest in studying with me but only attended once or twice before vanishing. They would then replicate my work under a different name, without giving any credit to the original creator. Brazilians seem to struggle significantly with acknowledging and validating others, regardless of their expertise or contributions.

My experience in Colorado was initially entirely different. The students who graduate from teacher training and began teaching independently in various locations and studios proudly identified themselves as practitioners of Kaiut Yoga. This open, committed, and mature attitude left a profound impression on me and brought me immense joy.

A few years later, when my student Yvonne Mosser learned that I was working on a project to license schools under the Kaiut Yoga brand, she approached me with great transparency,

"Look, I've been working with you for many years. Are you really going to start licensing schools under your brand?"

"Yes, I am!"

"In that case, I want to be the first! I want to carry your name!"

Yvonne met Francisco during the classes in Hotchkiss. She resided in Telluride, 108 miles (174 kms) to the south. With a small permanent population of 2,585 inhabitants (in 2023), Telluride serves as a microcosm of the broader Colorado experience described in this narrative.

When you position yourself on the main street, you are enveloped by buildings whose architecture evokes the legends and history of the American West's conquest, the epic advance to the new frontier. The famous New Sheridan Bar is a standout—a modern-day saloon steeped in Western lore. Some 300 buildings are listed as historical heritage sites, creating a palpable connection to a past when the Ute people also inhabited the region. Following this era, the town, then known as Columbia, was also the place of a mining boom of silver, gold, copper, zinc, and lead.

It was a time of prosperity that attracted not only prospectors but also adventurers of all kinds, as you can imagine. Notably, the infamous outlaw Butch Cassidy made his debut in large-scale crime here before teaming up with the Sundance Kid. The duo eventually fled to Patagonia down in Argentina and Bolivia, their exploits later immortalized by Robert Redford and Paul Newman in the 1969 classic western film. That iconic movie also featured the Oscar-winning song *Raindrops Keep Fallin' on My Head*, sealing their story into pop culture history.

Standing on the street today, you are greeted by the majestic expanse of the San Juan Mountains, a stunning segment of the Rocky Mountain range. This breathtaking view hints at the region's wealth of nature, adventure tourism, and alpine sports, including the renowned ski fields of nearby Mountain Village. Since 2007, this picturesque setting has also hosted the Telluride Yoga Festival. The annual four-day event attracts about a thousand participants and features lectures, performances, workshops, and activities led by esteemed yoga teachers. And now, with this vibrant setting in mind, we return to Yvonne, fully aware of the new universe that is opening for Francisco and his method.

I'm English and worked on cruise ships for four years, during which time I befriended a girl who had previously worked in Telluride, a place I had never heard of. Once, when we docked in New York, we rented a car to travel to California on vacation, intending to cross the United States from coast to coast. Midway through our journey, we decided to make a stop in Telluride. We arrived in the darkness of the night.

When I woke up the next morning, I looked around and thought, "Whoa! What place is this? Because it's wonderful!" We decided to spend the summer here instead of going to California. That's when I met John, whom I would marry six months later, in March 1981. John was nicknamed 'Duck' because of his duck-billed haircut.

In the first ten years of our marriage, we had no children, as planned. I learned to ski, we went hiking in the mountains, and we camped. The town was small and friendly. It was true love that kept me here, because we didn't have much money. John worked as a driver for a company, and I juggled multiple jobs, cleaning houses, taking care of children, walking dogs, and being a secretary.

Having been trained as a massage therapist during my time on the ships, I decided to work part-time in massage therapy after the birth of my first son, Clifford. Around that time, a German woman named Margot Pope, a yoga teacher from the Iyengar tradition, arrived in town. I began taking classes with her three times a week. Since there were more Iyengar teachers in Durango, 110 miles (175 kms) southeast of here, I started attending workshops there as well.

I had another son, Mitchell, and by the time my two children reached high school age, I was determined to become a yoga teacher. I completed a 500-hour training program accredited by the Yoga Alliance, well above the minimum requirement of 200 hours. When my teacher, Nancy Stechert, first mentioned Francisco and invited me to his course at the wonderful studio she had set up in Hotchkiss, a two-and-a-half-hour drive from here, I accepted. At that time, Francisco visited the studio twice a year, in January and July, having just started his first teacher training course.

The first time I attended his class his English was not good at all. But as soon as I placed my hands under the bolster at the beginning of the practice, I thought, "Oh, this is cool!" I immediately liked the practice and the teacher. I was already accustomed to yoga teachers with massive egos, constantly circling around and barking orders, completely contrary to what yoga should be. But Francisco was different. He was kind and good-natured. It was clear that he knew a lot and that his method was evolving.

Around that time, some people had opened the Telluride Yoga Center, where I was already working as a teacher. I invited Francisco to teach there, and it was an immediate success. I started with one class, but the space could only accommodate 36 people. Soon, I had to set up additional classes, and before long, I was opening one class after another.

But then, at a certain point, the owners of the place went behind my back and invited Francisco to offer a teacher training course. I was furious with these people. Francisco didn't know they were acting that way and were effectively cheating me. When he found out, he refused to go along with them. That's when I had the idea of opening my own space. Even so, I was already 62 years old and not a businessperson. How was I going to start a new career at this point?

Francisco encouraged and supported me a lot. When he came to Telluride, he stayed with us. I would sit at the table, work through the business numbers with a pencil, and show my husband, John, that Francisco knew how to manage money better than I did. In November 2017, we opened the first Kaiut Yoga studio in North America. I rented a beautiful space on the main avenue of the city. It was small, accommodating 20 to 22 yoga mats, but we received more people when Francisco visited. When that happened, I spread mats into the hallway through open doors, turning three usually separate spaces into an expanded class environment.

Francisco told me that I would have to choose between Iyengar and Kaiut Yoga to open the studio, saying it would be incompatible to work with both. What convinced me to choose Kaiut were the results I had experienced personally, especially with my sciatic nerve, and the improvements I observed in others. Although some of my students from my Iyengar days did not understand my change and did not follow me, most stayed. They, along with my new students, come and stay for the results. They notice how much the method improves their lives and how it helps them become more coherent and centered individuals.

A lot of people, when they first arrive to yoga, don't tell you everything. They don't mention their hip problem, or shoulder issue, or the things they've forgotten about. But after practicing for a while, one day they come to you, delighted, and say,

"Oh, my God! I had this neuropathy in my foot! And now it's better!"

The community here at the studio is very loyal. I have students who have been with me for a long time. Telluride isn't just a vacation spot. Many celebrities have winter or permanent residences here. Tom Cruise had a mansion here for many years, as did filmmaker Oliver Stone. Oprah Winfrey still does. Two-time Oscar-winning actor Hilary Swank has been my student, though I'm not sure when she'll be back after having twins in April 2023 at the age of 48. She loves Kaiut Yoga.

I have had students who are skiers, trail hikers, and people who do adventure tourism all over the world. Mature women, my age and older, often bring their husbands, family members, and friends. Younger people also attend. On average, people who in their 40s start to become interested in this type of work, often due to knee problems or changes in their mental process.

And hence, the high quality of the method and the genius of Francisco, which he shares with us in the teacher training, makes a significant difference and produces results. The magic lies in beginning our work with the nervous system. The way we open and close the practice is crucial because it creates a mental state that changes how the nervous system functions.

In the beginning, in Telluride, people were drawn to Francisco because of his charisma. However, many didn't appreciate the method, as they were accustomed to practicing yoga with the goal of achieving a beautiful body. They found the method too slow and expected a practice that left them sweating and immediately transformed. Consequently, only those who were ready to work on themselves truly appreciated the method.

Francisco continued to perfect his use of words, explaining the magic of the method—the meditation that arises and the process of getting to know yourself by going inside yourself. He became an even more talented speaker, honing his ability to effectively convey his points. He can take a student, clearly show what he wants, and then have everyone practice what he has just explained. His accent is no obstacle, and his good looks don't hurt either. Nowadays, his English is better than ours! He continues to evolve, never being repetitive, and always finding new ways to impact and engage people. He is highly sensitive, has a great sense of humor, and knows how to crack a joke at the right time.

This all resulted in Francisco creating a base of students and followers here in Colorado and beyond. It's not a cult, as some have called it, but a network of dedicated followers.

I am eternally grateful to Francisco for changing my life, for positively affecting both mine and my son Clifford's lives. He has helped me become a better person in my service to others and in my dedication to helping people. He has given us a career and has been a tremendous mentor and teacher to Cliff, providing my son with direction and openness that are truly blessings.

Cliff a certified teacher of the method and partner to his mother, alternates teaching classes with her at the Kaiut Yoga studio in Telluride.

At age 27, back in Telluride after some time away, I was trying to become an outdoor educator for young people. After high school, I realized that I don't fit the conventional professions. I abandoned the idea of going to a traditional college because my mind is more like that of an artist.

Listening to my heart and knowing that I wanted to somehow work in education, I spent a semester in Alaska taking the NOLS Outdoor Leadership and Nature Education course. There, I fell in love with mountaineering. I then spent another semester with NOLS in Mexico, focusing on sailing and sea kayaking. Returning to Colorado, I took two undergraduate courses in outdoor education and recreational leadership. I also got certified as an AGMA guide. However, upon completing this certification, I realized that I didn't want to be a guide. I didn't want to be a nanny for anyone in the mountains.

NOLS, the National Outdoor Leadership School, is an NGO based in Wyoming with campuses in various regions of the world, including, for a time, one in the Brazilian Amazon. On the other hand, AMGA, the American Mountain Guides Association, is an NGO based in Boulder that aims to lead in education, set standards, and advocate for the interests of these professionals.

The plan to return to Telluride and become an educator failed. I couldn't find my place and ended up working as a window washer. It was okay for me, climbing stairs and buildings, doing the whole job. However, considering myself highly qualified in mountaineering and wanting to pursue it further, I started climbing mountains. There are 52 mountain peaks over fourteen thousand feet [4260m] high in Colorado, many of which are around Telluride.

Mount Sneffels stands at 14,153 feet [4,315 meters] high. I took my climbing partner Garrett, and we drove 45 minutes from Telluride to get there. After a hike of about five miles [8 kms] to the base of the climb, we undertook roughly 2000 feet [610 meters] of technical, rope-assisted climbing to reach the halfway point of the peak. Then, we saw a storm approaching. It began to snow.

Then it's like, "okay, we're in a worse situation, we have to get out of here!"

We had rappelled down about 500 feet [150 meters] and were deciding whether to continue driving equipment into the ice or rocks to descend, as the conditions had changed drastically. Then I made a mistake. I slipped and fell. I was loose, no longer connected to the rope system. Garrett shouted,

"Self-arrest, self-arrest!"

Self-arrest is a mountaineering technique used to stop a slide or fall on snow or ice. One self-arrests by driving an ice axe, a similar piece of equipment, or one own hands or feet into the slope, using body weight for stabilization and friction, anchoring oneself to the surface you are sliding down or past, slowing or stopping the unwanted decent.

I attempted to self-arrest using my ice climbing tool, but it slipped out of my hand. I then tried to anchor myself with my left foot crampon, but it resulted in the most severe ankle sprain imaginable. I continued sliding and falling, my head snapping violently to the side. I struck my left leg against the mountain corridor, sustained head trauma, injuries to my C5 and C7 vertebrae, a bone bruise on my hip, a partial cut on my ear, and internal bleeding. I fainted.

Garrett thought I had died. But he climbed down to where he believed I had fallen. In the meantime, I regained consciousness and realized I was in a dire situation. I pulled on my lined emergency coat, crawled out of the snow and ice, and moved out of the avalanche danger zone. I descended into a field of rocks further down and could only crouch behind a boulder the size of a car before losing consciousness again.

Garret arrived at where I had fallen. He didn't see me there, but he found the trail of blood. He followed the trail and found me. He woke me up, made a quick assessment of my level of consciousness. He asked if I knew who I was, if I knew where we were. He realized that my level of consciousness was too low to think about a professional emergency rescue. He saw that I had a head injury and spinal injury. If he left me there to go for help, I would die. He made the decision to carry me with a spinal injury. He basically carried me out of there for five miles [8kms]!

I don't have much recollection of that part, likely because the trauma blocked my memory. But Garrett told me later,

"You knew you were at your worst, that you were all messed up, that we needed to get out of there. But it didn't help at all. You said, 'I can't do it anymore, I can't do it anymore!' And I said, 'you must get up, you must get out of this!'"

He took me to the hospital in Telluride, dropped me off in the emergency room, and called my mom. The staff provided basic care and fought to save my life, but there wasn't much more they could do. I needed specialized neurological care, but the storm made it difficult. They eventually managed to get me into an ambulance for a three-hour drive to a specialized emergency medical center in Grand Junction.

I woke up a day or two later, though I don't remember exactly. I went back to live with my mom and dad because I needed a lot of help, getting out of bed, using the walker, and going to the bathroom. I wore a cervical brace for five or six months. It was in this state that I met Francisco. When physiotherapy released me, I started doing Kaiut Yoga with my mom, four times a week. After three months, I experienced the spectacular results of the method. Essentially, I stopped feeling pain.

The doctors had told me that I had broken my neck in two places, but no one mentioned that I could have nerve injuries, which I did on the left side in my arm, hand, shoulder, and neck. But with yoga, I regained the mobility I was losing. This encouraged me to try climbing the mountains again. I thought, 'Wow, I'm cured!'

And I walked away from yoga...

I went back to my manual work of washing windows. As I did, the pain returned, all of it. The same patterns resurfaced. I sank into a cycle of drugs and alcohol, trying to avoid and numb the pain as much as possible. It didn't work. In fact, things got much worse. I hit rock bottom.

I had no idea, when wearing the orthopedic neck brace as I met Francisco, that I was on my way to landing in this work. Because I came out of the crisis when I returned to yoga, so I decided to take teacher training with him, in person, in Telluride. At Yvonne's studio! In my mother's studio!

I felt very privileged to have this intimate training experience with Francisco, as our group was just 25 to 30 people. In Boulder, the class would have been about 100 people, so it wouldn't have been as personal as it was here. I completed the 300-hour training, but I understand that this is a process of continuous education. I also took part in some additional activities with him in Boulder. I became a teacher and started teaching. As everything grew, I quit my job as a window cleaner. I am now a full-time, year-round Kaiut Yoga teacher, conducting nine classes a week in our studio.

I'm 33 years old now. I can't say that I'm completely free of pain, but I have a much different relationship with it. Pain is no longer my enemy or something to be avoided. It's more like my mind trying to communicate with me, signaling whenever there is something that needs my attention.

After everything that happened, I realized that Kaiut Yoga has become the foundation of my life in many ways. That's why I practice almost every day. I often say that the accident was the worst thing that happened to me, but it was also the best because it set me on this path.

Francisco's journey, mapped out in this non-linear narrative, was steadily broadening its horizons, charting paths to other destinations and evolving into new formats. It radiated from the original offerings in Hotchkiss, the activities in Boulder, and the inspiring teacher training program in Telluride. From the first school with Yvonne in the old mining town turned luxury tourist hub, developments would further unfold thanks to this dedicated and resourceful woman.

Yvonne's commitment to the method is evident through her participation in intensive periods of learning with Francisco in Curitiba, São Paulo, and two other international cities that you will soon discover. She possesses a charm and an innate ability to creatively navigate challenges—qualities that embody the Brazilian saying "dar um jeitinho," which means "to find a way." These strengths worked in tandem, allowing her to secure spots for at least two individuals in Francisco's fully booked events. These attendees, captivated by what they experienced, became instrumental pioneers in the further expansion of the Kaiut Yoga brand. These individuals completed training courses and went on to establish licensed schools in St Louis, Missouri, and Austin, Texas, marking further significant steps in the brand's growth, beyond Colorado.

Over time, more schools opened in Colorado, including Broomfield near Boulder, Durango near the border with New Mexico, and most eventually Denver. Boulder too would have its own dedicated school—with a second location in Longmont, 19 miles (31 kms) away—creating a significant base for expansion. On the East Coast, the first school would open in Bethany Beach, Delaware.

While the educational part of the work flourished smoothly, the same cannot be said of the commercial aspect and the business partnerships necessary to sustain it. Turbulence arose after takeoff, as this metaphorical aircraft—be it Boeing, Airbus, or perhaps more fittingly, Embraer of Brazilian ingenuity—gained altitude.

When Boulder started to stand out as a pivotal hub in our growth, a former student of mine, from Curitiba, who was living in Dallas, Texas, felt very moved by this success. She began to dream of setting up a school of her own. I supported it by licensing a school along the lines of Boulder, which is our ideal model.

From a certain point, however, the school entered a cycle of overspending, relying heavily on loans from individuals and banks.

She began marketing the work using images that had nothing to do with us, misrepresenting us, while continuing to use our brand. And then I realized that her approach had shifted into something different, something more ego-driven. She did not show the same common sense that everyone who works with us today has. The people who are with us today, really understand the method.

When the debts increased, she had a breakdown. Then she broke ties with us. She changed the brand, but in essence kept in the logo, making slight aesthetic changes to our encircled K logo from Kaiut Yoga. It looks slightly different, but it is unmistakably our K. She partnered with another individual, and from what I observed, their content was weak, lacking the depth and coherence that define our work.

Another situation in Canada, brought its own headaches and was quite controversial, though it did result in at least one positive outcome. This story revolves around a period when Francisco considered centering international operations in the northern neighbor of the United States. For a time, he held events there, including a teacher training course that even attracted students who had been following him in Colorado.

Yvonne:

I got a place for Heidi Philip from Toronto when she arrived wanting to study with Francisco, even though the class was already full. I didn't know her before. I just wanted to help. Soon, as a student, she managed to become Francisco's business partner. She started organizing many things behind the scenes, and it became clear that Francisco wanted someone to handle the business side so he could focus on his work as the talented teacher he is.

Early on, I saw that things were getting complicated between them on many levels, but I tried not to get involved because I had never had any issues with Francisco. He had always been sweet to me, and our work engagements had always been smooth. However, I observed that Heidi's management style was challenging, and her relationship with others, including with the company managing Francisco's work, was difficult.

One good thing, at least, came out of that situation. A group of European students who had taken the course in Toronto and then in the United States introduced a Dutchman to Francisco's work. He was so enchanted that he invited Francisco to conduct a teacher training course in Amsterdam. Yvonne, fully committed to her training process, attended the trainings in Canada and Europe.

I couldn't attend the first invitation due to scheduling conflicts. With so many invitations, I had to focus exclusively on teacher training and decline smaller events, even from places like Costa Rica, Mexico, New York, and California. Since the request from the Netherlands was for an experimental project for teachers, we agreed that I would send Ravi. It was his first international public presentation, a class for about 300 people. This experience was remarkable for him and led to a regular schedule of activities for teachers in the Netherlands.

The teacher training course I originally created was divided into three modules: "The Concept," the theory of method; "The Teaching Side," the pedagogical methodology; and "The Edge," a deep experience of practice. In total, it was an intensive 30-day course. Participants came not only from Holland but also from Germany, England, and Belgium.

As a result of this triple expansion in the United States, Canada, and Europe, growth occurred not only through exclusively dedicated studios but also through accredited teachers operating in these two countries, as well as in the Netherlands, Germany, Portugal, and South Africa. Naturally, Brazil will also be a focus of expansion, which will be discussed later in this narrative.

But back in Canada, trouble erupted.

Heidi had enticed me with the idea of expanding the method, with Toronto as the first location. However, she lacked understanding of entrepreneurship, business operations, and tax regulations. She had spent her entire career at a giant advertising company in a specific administrative role, making her highly technical but limited in business acumen. Her experience was that of a mid-level employee, accustomed to six weeks of vacation a year and seven-hour workdays. In contrast, I was used to working 12 to 15 hours a day. When I began to notice this discrepancy, it became clear that Canada, with its brutal bureaucracy, was one of the worst countries in the world for entrepreneurship. It had nothing in common with the United States.

When the need for a large volume of energy arose, she had nothing to deliver. When we raised investment and she took charge of managing the funds, she started off poorly, spending excessively. Things went wrong due to the unrestrained spending.

I pulled the brakes completely. I called her, but she didn't answer. I had been with her in person two days before. Her father, who I didn't know, was the one who eventually called me back. He said that she was depressed. Then things got heated. Because, how to have a partnership with someone who is getting unwell, and doesn't warn you?

She fabricated a bizarre conversation between me and her father. I ended the partnership, but all our money was tied up in a Canadian account. It took several months to resolve the situation, involving a complex process with Canadian law and a Canadian citizen. I had to start a formal process just to recover a fraction of what we lost. It was an absurd ordeal.

Ultimately, it was very liberating to realize that every time I attempted to manage or agreed to work with these individuals, who seemed impressive and proclaimed grand visions of taking over the world and securing funds, the outcomes were consistently problematic and contentious. They couldn't deliver and where actually leeches in the process.

I then had a conversation with Ravi.

"My place is in the classroom, where I can teach. That means far more to me than the consequences, you know? If everything falls apart, so be it. I'll be a happy beggar teaching yoga at Praça da Sé, the famous square with the Cathedral in downtown São Paulo. And that's okay. The rest is not my dream. If you want to expand, run this as a business, and grow it, that's up to you. It's not my talent. But if you want to pursue that direction, you are the one who can make it happen."

14

Here, There, and Everywhere

Telluride in Colorado and Gramado in Rio Grande do Sul hold a special place on Francisco's historical map, standing out as more than just popular tourist destinations. These towns share a unique allure that extends beyond the natural beauty of their mountainous landscapes. Both destinations are enriched by cultural events that infuse them with a special charm, creating a romantic atmosphere where nature, social elegance, and culture converge.

Though both towns have modest resident populations, they experience a significant influx of visitors drawn by this enchanting combination. Gramado is famed for its traditional film festival, while Telluride hosts both film and music festivals, along with the annual yoga festival. This blend of cultural vibrancy and scenic beauty cements their reputation as captivating tourist hotspots.

The scenery of Telluride is simply stunning. Towering aspen groves and majestic rock walls dominate the landscape. In the distance, the snow-capped peaks of the mountains offer breathtaking views in all directions. On sunny days, the sky is a brilliant blue, with pleasant temperatures, ranging between 65 to 70 degrees Fahrenheit (18 to 21 degrees Celsius).

The gondola—the only free public cable car transport in the entire country—whisks you from Telluride to the nearby Mountain Village, which stands 850 feet (259 meters) above town, in just 13 minutes. The hotels, with their architecture reminiscent of a charming alpine village, add to the picturesque setting.

Francisco would present at the Telluride Yoga Festival on multiple occasions over the years, joining a cast of dozens of renowned and prestigious teachers from all over the country. The festival became one more opportunity to exhibit his work, increasing the notoriety that had been gradually expanding since the initial courses and lectures, allowing his name to reach a wider audience.

Over the years he presented sessions that covered various themes, from introducing the method, "What is Kaiut Yoga?"; to the vast exploration of "What is Our Human Potential?"; to more technical topics, such as "Flexibility and Rigidity: Understanding the Restrictions and How they Develop."

In the 2015 event Francisco gained added publicity momentum thanks to a spotlight feature in *Yoga Journal*. The article by Melinda Dodd, Yoga Rebels: 5 Teachers Who Can Change What You Think of Yoga, highlights yoga's revolutionary nature and the conservative societal reactions it often provokes, from ancient India to B.K.S. Iyengar. She emphasizes that in the United States, yoga has broken free from its label as an alternative culture and is now firmly embedded in mainstream American society, with 21 million practitioners. She goes on to say that despite this, "some teachers still strike out in their own direction, challenging familiar rhetoric and provoking discussion about what yoga really is."

Dodd introduces five rebels, each making a significant impact on the American yoga scene with their provocative, transformative, and sometimes controversial, proposals. These innovations included mixing yoga and dance with hula hoops, combining performance yoga with Asian martial arts, integrating yoga with the physical and mental endurance practices of the U.S. Navy SEALs, and merging yoga with the evangelical Christian tradition through incorporating Bible readings into the practice, in contrast to the Bhagavad Gita of the Hindu tradition.

You might reasonably assume that Francisco would feel privileged to be included in this list of five emerging yoga innovators, pioneers shaping the future of the practice, right? I thought so too. But perhaps we need to reconsider our assumptions...

I have this thing that I adhere to: I never research what others are doing. I simply don't want to know. I need to maintain a sense of freedom in my mind, free from external influences, you know?

But in this case, I asked a student of mine to read the article before it was published so he could inform me about what these guys were doing. He spoke with the journalist, gained some access to the content, and did some research on who these people were. Then he came back to tell me

I felt embarrassed to be featured in that article. I found myself thinking, wow, this is great for brand visibility, but at the same time,

I'm ashamed my name is included among them... [laughter] These guys were really bad! It was all very Americanized, people mixing techniques, doing a lot of different things. They were just perpetuating the same mistakes that America was already making with yoga.

However, attending the Telluride Yoga Festival was an enjoyable experience. I realized that dealing with large audiences wasn't mysterious at all. Large audiences are just that, large. Participating in multiple events of the festival and other similar events proved to be quite interesting. These events are fundamentally simple. They are not merely platforms to showcase your work. They are stages to put on a show.

And this show is about creating an experience through sensations and speech. At the Festival, I noticed that there was something particularly good, light, and playful about it, making the experience delightful for everyone involved. Incorporating elements like lightness, good humor, and wit enriches your ability to bring a sense of presence to a lighter, more engaging territory.

For a moment, participating in events made me realize that I could make a professional living from it... if I wanted to. However, I quickly understood that this would never be a sign of success for me, internally. I had already observed an entire generation of teachers who made their living from events and workshops yet failed to deliver meaningful results to anyone.

The real show, the one where you reveal who you truly are, happens when you have just three students in the classroom. It occurs when you have worked with these three students over an extended period, allowing you to become a co-author in their journey and personal development.

The experience of lightness at events reinforced my understanding of its importance in the classroom. A stern environment is unhelpful as it fosters a lack of empathy. Students need to learn how to handle pain in a healthy way and build resilience to the everyday stresses of life, such as bad traffic, job pressures, and living in a polluted, violent city.

I began to understand that students needed to become resilient in every aspect of their lives. The class needed to be a controlled exercise in physical, mental, and emotional resilience. To achieve this, an environment of lightness is essential. It's crucial to convey to students that yoga is about equipping them to handle all aspects of life, including increased stress and whatever challenges may come their way.

And then an understanding was also born that would be consolidated much later, at the time of the COVID-19 pandemic. Deprived of physical presence with students and the ability to connect in person with hundreds of lecture attendees, I faced the challenge of delivering a large volume of content in a brief time. It was then that I realized the power of the teacher's voice. It became my Harry Potter wand.

The magic wand. Everything happens through the voice. Through intelligent guidance... the understanding of timing... and thoughtful inflection. It involves choosing a tone of voice that resonates with each student... so that they don't need to start up a discourse in their mind.

This is incredibly good. But while Harry Potter's magic wand is well-established in J.K. Rowling's books and the films, Francisco's wand is still navigating the subconscious realms of creative dreams, as seen in his early presentations at the Telluride Yoga Festival.

However, this brings us to an unexpected challenge in his broader creative mission—where the voice, though fundamental, is just one piece of a larger puzzle in developing his method. On one occasion, while Francisco was scheduled and announced as a guest teacher, an unforeseen issue arose while he was already en route. Unable to lead the event himself, he had to rely on his steadfast collaborator, Yvonne Mosser, to step in as his last-minute replacement.

I was beginning my work in Canada and had several events scheduled in the United States as well. As was customary, I flew to Miami, my usual connection point. I often stopped there for one or two nights during my American trips to mitigate the impact of the time difference.

On this trip, traveling alone, I followed my typical routine for when I was alone in Miami. I spent the night, visited some restaurants, and then continued my journey to Toronto. There, I delivered my lecture, visited a few places, and began to get a feel for the city.

On my return, I headed to Pearson International Airport to catch a flight to Denver. It was a major holiday in the United States, a hugely significant one. I had never seen an airport so full in my life, with queues stretching endlessly.

When I arrived at the immigration checkpoint, I was stopped, for reasons I didn't understand. I was stopped not by Canadian immigration, but by American immigration. The United States has their own immigration checkpoint inside Toronto's airport, allowing them to pre-screen passengers before they board flights to the U.S.

I sensed there was tension, though I couldn't pinpoint the cause, perhaps due to the holiday or other reasons. Despite having a valid American visa, they subjected me to more questions than usual. Ultimately, they prevented me from boarding my flight to Colorado, forcing me to travel straight back to Brazil.

United by strong commercial, cultural, social, and human ties, Canada and the United States form the third highest international pair in terms of air traffic volume between nations. As of 2023, there are an astonishing 441 daily flights, on average, between destinations in the two countries. Pearson Airport, Canada's largest, accounts for forty-one percent of these flights to its neighbor.

The United States' immigration checkpoint at the airport is the largest of the few such facilities the country has installed abroad. Its aim is to streamline immigration procedures for flights to the U.S., reduce congestion at American entry airports, and pre-screen for undocumented immigrants. According to civil rights advocates, it also serves to prevent the embarkation of refugees seeking the American dream of freedom and wealth.

You can now assess the magnitude and context of the problem Francisco encountered that day. Imagine the implication of being denied entry to the United States, and the blow it dealt to his growing work in North America. It was then that another ally entered the scene, to give a decisive hand at this critical moment. Carlos Gloger.

Carlos:

I met Francisco when I was 28 years old. At the time, I suffered from scoliosis, hip pain, and significant shoulder pain due to work-related tension. As a practicing lawyer, these issues were particularly troubling. I sought his help at the insistence of my wife, Lorenza. Within three weeks of practice, the pain caused by everyday tension disappeared. Our student-teacher relationship evolved into a great friendship, to the point where I often cooked for him and his family at my house on weekends, or my family and I visited his home. Our relationship grew into an ultra-close friendship and included business support, with me acting as his lawyer.

Later, an exceedingly difficult moment came when he went through a separation in his marriage. I got along well with his wife too and wanted to help mediate the divorce. However, it turned out to be a disaster. It was one of the biggest mistakes I made in my life, and I almost lost our friendship over it. I lacked the professional maturity to realize that I shouldn't have put myself in that situation. I stepped down as his lawyer, and he then hired another attorney, which was the right move, as I was no longer able to help.

Amidst this crisis, I was his partner in the United States, and we had plans to start a business together. However, things began to fall apart. My role was to make things happen there, as Francisco has always been focused on teaching and less on external affairs. He has always needed a lot of support in this regard.

I arranged an event in the United States, which was supposed to be his first of the summer that year. However, he decided to go to Canada first.

"Why are you going to Canada, man?"

"It's a new project. I'm going to teach some weekend classes, while you take care of things in the United States."

I was a little pissed.

"Gee, we're barely starting the business, and now you're branching out to Canada! But, okay, okay, we'll talk later!"

It was during his trip from Canada to the United States that he was stopped by immigration. This was like throwing cold water on our U.S. business plans!

During this tumultuous period, our friendship was super shaken. He had once given me a photo from his trip to Tibet, and I always teased him,

"You didn't go to Tibet at all! You went to Marumbi Peak, near Curitiba! I've never seen a picture of you in Tibet."

After a while, he finally gave me a photo of him in front of some landmark there,

"Here's proof that I went to Tibet!"

"Okay!"

I kept the photo.

Then, amid our crisis, I invited him for coffee at Prestinaria, this famous bread house in Curitiba. I put the photo of Tibet on the table:

"Look, I'm here. I want to preserve our friendship. But if things continue the way they are, they will go to shit! So, let's separate as business partners, and I'll step down as your lawyer."

I continued to practice yoga regularly, attending classes as usual. For the first six months, we kept our distance. Gradually, we started to reconnect. It took about two or three years for our friendship to fully recover to the way it was before.

Let's take a step back to the past—and then forward again to the future. Once more, we return to Colorado. This time, the destination is Boulder. A new time, a new cycle.

After Yvonne's school opened in Telluride, a trio of students approached me. They also wanted to start their own business and generate their own revenue, but with a direct relationship with me. They sought a brand license. For me it was a connection to a content-producing source, and validation and promotion of the brand. This trio would eventually open the first Kaiut Yoga school in Boulder.

Kristin Savory has short dark brown hair and a lively expression. She exudes a certain aura of physical energy, akin to someone who practices sports. And she speaks with the quick, agile rhythm typical of women of action.

I met Francisco when my son Henry was two years old, and my daughter Nora was six. Henry's delivery was an emergency cesarean section. The births of my two children left me in significant pain for a long time. Nora left me with back pain that I was somewhat able to manage. However, Henry's case was more challenging. By the end of the day, I could no longer walk if I had to climb stairs. I had to drag my left foot. The pain started in my back, radiated down my leg, and into my left foot. Despite being an acupuncturist and having a background as an athlete—I had run in my school days—I couldn't control it.

I was receiving massages from a chiropractor and having sessions with an acupuncturist friend of mine. On a scale of zero to ten, my back pain was at an eight. After the sessions, the pain would decrease to a three, but the relief only lasted for a week.

A friend of mine then told me,

"There's this guy from Brazil coming to Boulder to teach yoga classes for two weeks, three times a day. I don't know if he will help you, but I think you should give it a try and maybe even study with him a bit."

I decided, "Okay, I'll take a class and see what happens."

So, I went! And it was difficult! The room was crowded, and people were moaning in pain! The class was very intense.

Nevertheless, somehow, I felt better afterward. I decided to attend as many classes with Francisco as possible while he was here. I arranged for babysitters for the children and found a way to make it work so I could attend the classes.

And then my pain went down from an eight to a three. But since I was used to temporary relief, I thought, "okay, let's see if it lasts." And you know what happened? I was pain-free for five months. When Francisco returned six months after I first practiced with him, I attended as many classes as I could.

That was 12 years ago. Since then, I have had no more pain, if I practice Kaiut Yoga.

For about two years, I kept the practice to myself. I was exhausted, you know? I was a young mother with two small children, a husband, and a career as an acupuncturist, all of it. I was so happy to have found a practice where I felt like I was finally taking care of myself, rather than always focusing on the kids, my husband, clients, and the community. I felt much better in my body. Because of the positive results from yoga, I stopped needing massages, acupuncture, that kind of thing.

Then I started to try a few things with my clients. I'd think, oh, let's see what happens if I do sukhasana before applying the needles, or what if they turn their head and I give the client a massage? They would come back, asking for more and wanting to know what I had done in the last session.

It became clear to me that it had nothing to do with acupuncture. It had to do with the fact that I had brought some of the elements I had learned in yoga.

Still, I wasn't entirely convinced. I felt like I had an excellent job and a profession I loved, so I thought I would keep things as they were. But after about five years, I started to think differently. I wanted to make a bigger impact on the world. In my community, I realized I could reach more people by teaching yoga. Although I had specialized in acupuncture, particularly in working with women and hormone issues, I asked myself if I could achieve better results with yoga. It was clear right away that I could.

There is something else very dear to my heart. When I started as an acupuncturist, I never wanted people to depend on me. It seemed unethical to me. I wanted to empower people to take care of themselves. In yoga, I found an avenue to fulfill this perspective. Of course, I use my words and share some of my knowledge, but I primarily teach people to connect with themselves and use their own bodies. And that's a wonderful resource.

In my 21 years of acupuncture practice, I've never had a client say, "Kristin, I had a migraine last night, I rubbed point 36 on my stomach, and point 62 on my bladder, and I felt better."

However, every month, several students come to me and say, "I wasn't feeling well, so I put my legs up on the wall and did some things I remembered from the last class. Now I feel much better."

It's extraordinary. You have a system you can use for your own benefit, health, and vitality.

When I made this connection, I had no more doubts. This is what I want to commit my life to: working with many people on yoga mats, rather than just one person on the table. I enrolled in Francisco's teacher training, which led to a supportive relationship that gave me the confidence to pursue this path. However, I knew I couldn't do it alone. I wasn't interested in being someone's employee. I wanted to be a leader. This desire led me to consider opening a yoga studio. That's when I crossed paths with Darvin and Craig.

It was kind of funny. The three of us were taking Francisco's teacher course. I barely knew Darvin and had only spoken to him briefly a couple of times. During a break, he approached me and said,

"Hey, I want to tell you something. I'm thinking about the idea of maybe opening a yoga school in Denver."

I looked at him and replied,

"Well, why would you want to open in Denver? Why not do something closer?"

He hesitated for a moment and then asked,

"What are you thinking?"

I said,

"Why not open a school with me?"

It was like that. Then we had many conversations about the subject. And there was a certain impression on my part that it would be better to have three partners at the beginning, rather than just two. I had known Craig for much longer, we had done a lot of training together, I feel a close connection with him. He's like a younger brother of mine.

We went to lunch, on one day during training. I remember very well the bagel we were eating, when I said,

"Hey, what are your intentions with Kaiut Yoga? Would you be interested in opening a school?"

The three of us approached Francisco and opened Kaiut Yoga Boulder.

Like with any new beginning, whether in business or in life, challenges await around the first corner.

Our biggest challenge was not having our own space. But that was okay. We really wanted to start from scratch. We began in a synagogue, the Jewish Nevei Kodesh Congregation. They rented us a space where we could store our things, but we had limited options for times and dates due to their activity calendar. Still, it fit within our budget. We started with about 15 lessons a week and had Francisco as a special guest for his intensive classes whenever he was in town.

Then our student membership grew rapidly. In six months or so it became clear that we needed a bigger space and more time options. We found a suitable space at the Meadows Shopping Center, but we had to do a major renovation. This took a year or so.

In September 2019, we inaugurated the new space with a fantastic party that Francisco attended. It was beautiful, incredible! And shortly after, in January 2020, we held Francisco's first teacher training course, attracting around 115 students or so.

And then, the pandemic arrived. It hit us hard. We had to enter the digital world as quickly as we could. We navigated that time quite successfully and at the end of the day, we grew. In 2022 we opened our second location in Longmont, close to Boulder.

Francisco sees the Boulder school as a strong partner for expanding the brand abroad, much like Yvonne Mosser's school in Telluride. However, as a faithful representative of this model, Kristin has also witnessed less-than-ethical actions from opportunists. She has experienced the darker side of human nature that often accompanies success stories, especially in a capitalist and competitive society.

Here's the thing: Francisco is a genius, and the method is fantastic, but like anywhere there are a people in the field of yoga with ill intentions and motivations. Many times, I've seen people appropriating elements of his work. This might be a very American thing, though I'm not sure if it happens in Brazil too. People take aspects of his method and believe they can do it better than he can, thinking they fully understand his approach. There's a lot of ego involved, particularly from some teachers, and then things can completely fall apart.

Francisco has worked with many people in roles similar to mine, but I think our partnership works because none of us—Craig included, while he was with us—never wanted to replace Francisco. After all, he is the genius behind the method. We simply want to learn from him, with no other desire.

Craig was instrumental in jointly developing an innovative project with Francisco.

The project was incredibly successful. It was a series of podcasts that I called Reframing Yoga. *The podcasts aimed to reinterpret yoga within a broader health context, as proposed by the method. I studied various podcasts from around the world, identified some key inspirations, and, after thorough research, we launched our series very successfully. Craig's capabilities were invaluable in this endeavor.*

The series began in partnership with the Colorado Sleep Institute in Boulder, a clinical center specializing in sleep disorders. Over 11 episodes between August 2021 and May 2022, Francisco, with his improving English skills, often starred as the co-host alongside Craig. In a talk show format, they welcomed special guests to discuss several topics. When Francisco was absent, Craig ran the show seamlessly.

The episodes covered enriching topics like mental health and breathing, symmetry and adaptability, the nervous system and sleep, sleep disorders and insomnia, and understanding the mind-body connection in sleep. The series featured insightful dialogues with experts such as Adam Wertz, co-founder of the Institute, and Ellen Stothard, the director of research and development at the Institute, who has a PhD in physiology and neuroscience. Additionally, the series included testimonies from individuals with extensive experience in unconventional health paths, always seeking to find points of connection with the method.

We tried to do an episode every 15 days. But Craig didn't have much time and my schedule was tight. We were losing rhythm and fluidity, and the content became inconsistent. Then we had to stop doing it. But I really liked this work.

Darvin Ayre brought to the group his experience as a professional familiar with the business world, alongside his unconventional approach as an educator and consultant. He had been involved in programs related to human development and health processes throughout his life. This background helped him quickly recognize the value and visionary and transformative nature of Francisco's method. However, fully understanding the scope of the work took some time.

I worked for about 15 years with Outward Bound, a network of outdoor experiential learning schools, in mountain and desert programs across Colorado and Utah. I also had international assignments in Hong Kong, Australia, New Zealand, Africa, and Europe. The organization operates 35 schools worldwide. Additionally, I directed rehabilitation programs for individuals with alcohol and drug problems, worked with Vietnam War veterans suffering from post-traumatic stress disorder, and led adult recovery programs.

After leaving, I became a consultant. I have provided services to the Soros Foundation, owned by mega-investor George Soros, in Eastern Europe; to the National Institutes of Health in Great Britain; and to large health care organizations in North America, such as Kaiser Permanente and the American Association of Hospitals. I mean, I've always been involved in human development and the transformation of people.

Despite loving my work with these organizations and the people within their communities—I continue to chair one of Outward Bound's boards—it was finding the method and taking my current position at the school that marked the pinnacle of my interests and career. With Kaiut Yoga, I feel we are truly transforming people's lives. I can teach them and do an excellent job without fostering dependence. I'm not handing out pills or offering a checklist of ten improvements or a perfect meditation routine. Instead, I help them discover their own abilities to flourish. This is what I love! It's also what I see evolving in my own body and mind.

I've always been a trail runner and a cyclist, which kept me in good shape. But in 2010, I experienced horrible sciatic pain. I found some relief with yoga, but it was a different, rather dull practice. Then, in 2016, I discovered Kaiut Yoga. Within a couple of weeks, I felt something different happening, particularly in relation to another pain I was experiencing.

I have a wood stove here at home and a big truck. After coming home from a class in the afternoon, I had to take a load of firewood from the truck to the backyard to fuel the stove. I thought, this is going to hurt like hell! I'll pay the price for this tomorrow. However, in the morning, I woke up feeling great! This piqued my interest in the method. Over the next few months, I practiced regularly and discovered that Kaiut Yoga was not only beneficial for my physical body, but it also brought significant changes to my nervous system.

Craig and I were already friends, and we attended some of Francisco's classes together. I really enjoyed Francisco's teaching. When the teacher training course was announced, I initially thought I couldn't participate because my consulting work required a lot of travel. I didn't think I would have the time. However, two weeks before the course started, I realized there was no way I could miss it. I wanted to understand what was happening here. During the course, I had that pivotal conversation with Kristin, leading to the story you now know.

The most important thing I want to highlight here: until a couple of years ago I had no idea of the depth and power that this work delivers. From the beginning of the practice, I realized that my body was understanding more and feeling more. But it took me a while to realize that my nervous system and my thought patterns that shaped how I interact with the world, were changing. Only then did I get that, "wow, this is big!"

This is the beauty of Francisco's work. The body is a natural healing system, and we are just starting to understand this. Much of what we need to do is simply to close our minds to other preconceived notions of how we should heal ourselves. In my years of working with large healthcare organizations, I have led teams of outstanding professionals, including cardiovascular surgeons and specialists from various fields. I often heard stories about how the methods of conventional health systems frequently fail.

What I have understood from the method is that we can access this inner source of healing. Pain serves as a wonderful window into our deeper selves and source of healing.

Now, at 69 years old, I have a doctor who I see. He is the head of the complementary medicine area at Kaiser Permanente in Colorado. He monitors me for occasional pain in my right hip, left knee, and shoulder. I told him,

"I'm not going to have surgery. Who cares about this pain? It's nothing!"

The doctor examines me and says,

"No, that's fine. You're fine, really. Just keep doing what you're doing."

And what am I doing? Kaiut Yoga!

Am I going to retire now that I'm 69?

No! I might stop doing some things later, but I feel quite young, and even a bit immature. I'm always curious, you know? I love adventure and learning new things. That doesn't mean I'm not a bit stiff in body or rigid in thought sometimes. But through this work, I observe my body, recognize my patterns, and notice everything that is moving and changing. I see the progression in my own development as a human being.

This is what I love about the method. My motivation feels limitless, like the sky is the limit.

I became friends with Francisco and have traveled to Brazil many times to attend his events. This work is incredibly powerful. Francisco is a genius, and although I try not to inflate his ego too much—and even poke fun at him about it—he truly is in a category of his own.

I have always worked with fantastic people, excellent educators, who speak to integrating body and mind. They are incredible at understanding the intersection between the two.

Francisco understands this, but he's doing something more. He's delivering at a level of movement. He comprehends people's personalities through movement, understands their nervous systems, and knows how they tend to respond. This intricate understanding, woven together, surpasses everyone else. I've never seen anything like it. There may be other teachers out there with similar abilities, but I don't know them, and I'm not looking to find out.

What I do know is that I feel fortunate, because this work has helped me so much. If I can continue to evolve as a good teacher, I believe I can help bring this work to more people.

This definitive take-off in the United States—from Telluride to Boulder—marks a turning point in Francisco's story and the method. Meanwhile, in Brazil, it was Gramado that would become the gateway for expansion.

15

Four Noble Truths and Yoga in Serra Gaúcha

The identity of a group of people emerges from a complex interplay of psychological and archetypal processes, drawing from both real history and fictional narratives. These elements combine to create representative models of the collective soul, expressing the essence of that community. For the people of Rio Grande do Sul, the iconic image of the "gaúcho" often comes to mind.

In Porto Alegre, the capital of the state, the Laçador Statue stands as a powerful symbol of this identity. This bronze monument, towering fourteen and a half feet high (4.45 meters) and weighing nearly four tons, was crafted by sculptor Antônio Caringi. It captures the quintessential elements of gaúcho culture through the figure of a "pilchado"—a traditional gaúcho figure dressed in customary attire. The figure embodies the countryside horsemen of the pampas, the protectors of cattle, who wear classic "bombacha" trousers that are wide-legged and buttoned at the ankles. Other key cultural symbols surround him, including "chimarrão" (yerba mate tea), the criollo horse, and the quero-quero bird.

Tradition associates the gaúcho man with idealized masculine qualities such as courage, physical strength, and virility. While these traits can be beneficial for everyone, they often mask the darker aspects of this ideal, namely, violence and machismo, which are harmful. The thin line that separates virtue from excess is akin to a sharp blade, precarious and dangerous to navigate.

The gaúcho woman, on the other hand, is associated with strength of character, often combined with tenderness. This image has been preserved and celebrated in history and the arts, portraying women who resisted submission in a predominantly conservative and paternalistic society. Figures like Anita Garibaldi in historical records, Ana Terra in Érico Veríssimo's literature (*O Tempo e O Vento*), and Anahy in Sérgio Silva's film (*Anahy de las Misiones*) exemplify this resilient spirit.

An underlying thread in the lives of all genders—men, women, and others—is a universal challenge: none of us are perfect, and we are all here to evolve. What unites us is the field of suffering that spares no one. Our suffering is often the push of existence that kicks us into action. It is often a push based in love, even if it doesn't seem like it. Whether gaúchos or gaúchas, cowboys or cowgirls, in Brazil or America, this shared experience binds us all.

Camila Moscarelli, a Kaiut Yoga teacher in Gramado, an icon of the method in the state, owner of two licensed schools, one in the city and the other in neighboring Canela, belongs to the lineage of strong-willed women from Rio Grande do Sul.

One day, Francisco said to me,

"Camila, I want to make Gramado a Boulder. The same thing I have there, I want to have here. This will be my Boulder in Brazil."

I responded,

"I want that too! Let's do this together!"

Professionally, I have always gotten along very well with Francisco. However, he has his demands and his unique way of doing things. When we started, I noticed that he had a certain ease in cursing others. But when he tried to curse me, I had difficulty understanding it... [*laughter*]

After a long time of working together, I noticed that Ravi was trying to get a little closer to Francisco. It was very much a father and son thing. One day, I finally questioned Francisco,

"Who are you going to leave your intellectual heritage to? Are you going to keep it all to yourself? Are you going to let Ravi drift away, indifferent to your work? You must pass it on to someone! It can't die with you."

I'm not sure if my words had any influence, but after a while, Ravi came here, and we started working together on the events we organized. It was super cool. We had to adjust some things and improve a lot, continuously polishing our efforts. Eventually, they both realized that things were growing on this side, and the events here demanded more attention and a more professional and elaborate approach.

Initially, they didn't use social media for promotion that much. They had a student who helped with a blog, handling some of the digital aspects. But that was it. So, I contributed by actively promoting through my Instagram and Facebook, inviting my followers to attend the lectures and courses.

We were breaking attendance records one after another, with up to 75 students in a single room. Francisco created new versions of the courses, attracting participants from São Paulo and even the United States. Initially, the courses were aimed at students looking to enhance their practice with a therapeutic focus. Then came the teacher training program. The courses reached a level of acceptance that drew a very diverse audience, including many who wouldn't typically attend yoga events.

The journey to reach this point was arduous. Much had to change before Camila could contribute to the expansion of the method and play the pivotal role she holds in this story. It all began long ago with a beginning that was more than dramatic. It was tragic.

I was born in Cachoeira do Sul, in the interior of the state. When I was two years old, my family moved to Porto Alegre. We were very close to my aunt Sonia Beatriz Schmidt, my mother Maria Aparecida's sister. When I decided to move out and live on my own at 18, Aunt Sonia trusted me and rented me an apartment. We became incredibly close. Tragically, there was a car accident, and she, my uncle Rogério, and my eight-year-old cousin Vinícius lost their lives. Only my two-and-a-half-year-old cousin, Vitória, survived.

That moment made a thousand things explode in my head. Why are we alive? What are we doing here? It propelled me into a deep search for answers. Until I found Buddhism.

I went on to study with Lama Rinpoche at the Buddhist temple in Três Coroas, participating in practice sessions and retreats. This experience introduced me to more people in the realm of complementary therapies, an area I was already familiar with due to my father, Rudimar, who is a homeopath and acupuncturist. My mother, Maria, came from the fitness world, competing in bodybuilding. She always exposed us to healthy eating, including macrobiotics. Their influence was incredibly inspiring in terms of both food and body care. The natural wellness universe had always felt like it was courting me, and I was equally drawn to it.

When I discovered spirituality, it led me to reevaluate how I was using my body. This opened a universe of questions about my physical practices. People started mentioning yoga to me repeatedly, and eventually, I attended a class with a friend.

And when I left the class... wow! Dear yoga, I missed you! How did we stay apart for so long? This is what I want to do with my life! Yoga!

My vow was always to free people from suffering. I just didn't have the right tool. The death of my dear family members made me realize that everyone shares a common bond: we are all connected by suffering and the pursuit of happiness. I understood that it wasn't just me who was suffering. Everyone, in some way, is suffering. I wanted to liberate people from the ignorance of suffering.

The teachings of the Buddha supported everything I was feeling, adding structure and clarity to my thoughts. However, I still lacked a clear direction for my life. After the death of my family members, I delved into Japanese medicine, took courses in flower essences and massage therapy. When I discovered yoga, it had a profound impact. It moved my body and calmed my mind. The practice seemed to align with my needs. Yet, I soon realized that yoga wasn't a universal tool that worked for everyone, which was a source of great frustration for me for a long time.

Camila lived with this frustration, yet she persisted in exploring every style of yoga she could. She took courses in Porto Alegre, studying hatha yoga, ashtanga, and practicing flow yoga. When she discovered Iyengar yoga, she felt a deep connection. It was the form that truly resonated with her heart. She dove in completely, both head and heart.

During this time, Camila began a romantic relationship in Gramado, which led her to move to the city. She continued practicing yoga until her teacher, Lorita Festa, expressed a desire to change her work pace. Lorita offered Camila the chance to take over her classes in Canela. This marked the beginning of Camila's career as a yoga teacher, which received an extraordinary boost in the following years. She taught yoga at the luxurious Kurotel, a renowned clinical spa in Gramado, considered one of the best in South America.

Camila's talent for mobilizing people, forming and sustaining networks, and promoting events soon became evident. She emerged as an efficient promoter of Iyengar yoga, organizing events and workshops that featured renowned teachers. Concurrently, she continued her education by attending courses with prominent figures in São Paulo, Florianópolis, and Porto Alegre. As a natural result of her determined efforts, Camila eventually became the owner of a yoga school with two locations, one in Gramado and the other in Canela.

This deep involvement with yoga unfolded alongside the spiritual support she found in Buddhism. Camila admits that her move to Gramado was influenced not only by her relationship with Eduardo but also by her desire to be near the Chagdud Gonpa Khadro Ling Buddhist temple. Founded by the Tibetan monk Chagdud Tulku Rinpoche, the temple is located in nearby Três Coroas.

In Buddhism, Camila found the spiritual support she needed to grapple with the central issue of human suffering, which had deeply affected her. This is encapsulated in the essence of Buddha's teaching, the Four Noble Truths. These truths outline the path to liberation that Prince Siddhartha Gautama, who became the Buddha, presented to humanity: the truth of suffering, the origin of suffering, the cessation of suffering, and the path leading to the cessation of suffering.

Yet, Camila still sought a way to fulfill her life's purpose, deeply influenced by Buddhism: to contribute in her own way to the collective challenge of facing human suffering. She couldn't fully commit to Lama Rinpoche's unrealized project of establishing a support service for people in the terminal phase of life, a hospice offering palliative care. While volunteering at the temple during retreats was valuable, it wasn't sufficient. Nor did her time living in an ecological community near the temple provide the fulfillment she sought.

It wasn't until Camila met Francisco and discovered Kaiut Yoga that she found a path toward greater fulfillment. However, the road to these transformative encounters was anything but smooth—it was marked by, let's say, a few explosive moments along the way.

In 2013, I became pregnant. Professionally, I was doing very well with many students and life was unfolding beautifully. However, I suddenly began to question how the Iyengar method was being taught in the West. I started to re-evaluate the practice as it was happening here. I wished people could better manage the small stresses of life and rise above the ignorance of trivial sufferings; you know? Oh, one moment, I'm here, super happy...then, I get a not-so-pleasant phone call... and suddenly... life feels horrible because of something so small...

Pregnancy made me think... something... the presence of the spirit growing inside me made me question if I was on the right path. "Is this really what I want to do? The tool is yoga, but is it the right one?" I felt so frustrated. People were aging alongside me, students who had been with me for many years. Yet, "look at the hips of this woman. They haven't changed, still rigid. And the neck of that other person, still the same issues. My God, I think I might need to stop doing yoga!"

I didn't want to chant the mantras anymore. I no longer wanted to engage with the images. I took a bag, placed everything related to Hindu and Tibetan traditions, including photos of deities and messages from masters, into it. Then I closed it all in a chest.

Amid this difficult period, the name of Francisco began to ring in her ears and appear before her eyes through unexpected and intertwined paths. A girl from Curitiba, Fabíola Almeida, who had been working in Gramado for a time, once spoke to her about an incredible and innovative teacher from Paraná. A copy of *Yoga Journal Brasil* landed in her hands, featuring an article about this remarkable teacher with more than a thousand students. Even a client at Kurotel gifted her a book, inside which was Francisco's business card...

As time rolled on, her son Zion continued to grow while still nursing at a year and a half old. Then, one day...

The cell phone rang. It was Fabi. She had returned to Curitiba. She said that she had four modules left to complete a two-year training course with Francisco.

"I talked to my teachers about you. They said you can come and join this weekend's workshop. You will be our guest."

I replied,

"Oh, that's cool."

Fabi typically spoke to me in a very Zen way that didn't really touch my heart. I didn't want to go there or get to know Francisco's work. But this time, I thought, "oh, she has some energy about this!" She followed up, talked to the teacher, and called me at the last minute. It was a Monday, and the workshop would be on Friday of that same week.

I decided to go. I prepared milk for my son, got a ticket, and called aunt Lu to take care of Zion. My husband didn't like my sudden departure! [*laughter*] I think it shook the marriage a bit. You know how it is!? You let go of the child and run away! Because it's my life, for God's sake. It's a calling. My son, I'm sorry, but Mom has to go. You chose this mother. And this mother is crazy—for yoga! So, there I went.

When I arrived early in Curitiba, I set foot inside the room at the back of the Batel school. No one had arrived yet. I looked around and felt something friendly. I know this energy; I know this place.

I calmed down, completed the workshop, and began taking part in the next modules. I took their next training courses and never stopped. I got to know the method and thought, "I need to share this with my people! I need to bring this to my students, to help so-and-so, and to reach such and such person." I thought through all the people in my circle. Reflecting on my fellow teachers and friends, I realized that while we had a lot of goodwill, we weren't truly delivering yoga. I thought, "I had never truly delivered yoga to anyone!"

You might assume that Camila, being impulsive and falling in love with the new method she had just encountered, would then abandon all her activities with Iyengar yoga. Well, not quite...

In the meantime, after completing my third module of Francisco's course, a renowned Iyengar teacher came to give a workshop that was packed with attendees. I made a point of collaborating and invited many colleagues. Because I was always teaching Iyengar classes in various places in Rio Grande do Sul, many people who knew me showed up. The teacher was a colleague from the training course I had taken with the renowned teacher Kalidas Nuyken in São Paulo.

There I was, sitting cross-legged and such, when the teacher started singing a mantra in a voice that didn't seem like hers. It felt like everything froze for me in that moment. I looked at her from the corner of my eye and thought, "why is she chanting this mantra that no one knows?" I glanced at the people around me, sitting with poor posture... "What circus is this? This is not yoga, for God's sake! We are destroying our bodies. This can't continue. I need to bring real yoga to my people."

I told Francisco about the experience. His response,

"Why did you do that? Why did you go to the workshop in the first place?"

"Because I need to understand what is different between your yoga and Iyengar's. I had several insights during the workshop and realized I wasn't really doing yoga. But I need to understand more. There are similarities here—the bolster is the same, the strap is the same, the block and the wedge are the same. But what's different? I need to understand."

I felt that Francisco, quite energetically, took me by the hand and explained things in a way that I could understand. He put me in situations in the classroom in a more objective manner. He invited me to go with him in the courses and workshops he gave to teachers, using these opportunities to point out comparisons and differences between the two practices.

One of the great distinctions that became clear to me was that Kaiut Yoga does not focus on body alignment because it understands the impact alignment can have on the body. Adjusting positions and aligning in Iyengar practice can conceal blockages even more, making them invisible to the brain.

I then understood that the method alleviated the deep pain in my soul. The pain of human suffering due to ignorance. It calmed me because I realized that this method was a tool that resonated deeply with my Buddhist views.

How did Francisco experience the arrival of this student—one who was deeply respectful of all masters and teachers due to her Buddhist upbringing, yet also critical and questioning?

Camila has a naturally unifying and magnetic personality. She talks a lot with everyone, and people listen to and respect her. She brought many people to the first courses held in partnership with her in Gramado, people who would never have taken the chance to enter an unknown place if it weren't for Camila. They found the unique content that the method offers.

Among them was Evelise Pisani from Caxias do Sul, the daughter of one of the pioneers of yoga in Brazil and owner of the school she inherited from her mother. When Evelise got to know the method, she couldn't believe it could be so good. She wanted to see what other teachers in Rio Grande do Sul and São Paulo found most interesting. She returned to Camila and said:

"This guy cannot be real! This method is very good!"

From then on, it was one step after another, becoming increasingly connected with me. A very beautiful and strong story of transformation.

When I conducted the first teacher training course in Rio Grande, in partnership with Camila, I witnessed the birth of something special. It reminded me of what had happened in Hotchkiss, a kind of grassroots movement, with people leaving the capital to take the course in a more distant, rural area in search of knowledge. From this emerged a very solid, mature, and respectful approach from the people of Rio Grande towards my work, a level of engagement I had only seen before in the United States. There is a unique chemistry between the method and the people of Rio Grande do Sul that is truly special.

I noticed a pattern that parallels how gaúchos are renowned for exporting talent to universities and institutions across Brazil. Take Leandro Karnal, for instance—a distinguished historian, writer, lecturer, and one of the most influential contemporary thinkers in the country. Many like him have roots in the interior of Rio Grande do Sul, and from there, their influence spreads across Brazil. This dynamic spirit seems to resonate deeply with the philosophy and reach of the method.

In those first courses, I realized that the students in Rio Grande do Sul were very capable of listening. They were not tainted by prejudices or by the American commercial yoga that had captivated São Paulo. They didn't follow the carioca fads—the typical fanfare lifestyle of Rio de Janeiro—and hadn't bought into the American trends. However, they were lacking in information, and I wanted to provide that information in a human way. I aimed to connect and deliver to real people, after all. Additionally, there was a rich tradition in the south within the history of Brazilian yoga, names that did excellent work but were never recognized on a national level. I came to understand that the human potential in Rio Grande do Sul was very different.

All my trips there, even amidst my numerous international travels, became very pleasurable. I learned to relax, have fun, and enjoy the bonus of sharing the method. I became very good friends with Camila, and her new partner is my friend Leandro. I often tease him, saying he's the only gaúcho I know who doesn't know how to make barbecue.

There is an energetic match between my work and the Buddhist communities, much like in Boulder. I had very interesting conversations there with people from Naropa University and the local Buddhist community. Similarly, I felt a clear energetic alignment in the mountains of Rio Grande do Sul. Although I am a Buddhist, but not an extremely practicing one.

I see a simple yet important spontaneous connection between some precepts of Buddhism and my work, things that make a lot of sense. For instance, the idea that we are here to learn and evolve. From the moment we are born, a feeling of separation between mind and body arises. This leads us to understand the mental continuum that transcends incarnations. I realized that there is a very Buddhist aspect to yoga, which involves meditation, body practices, and breathing techniques.

I realized that there was a gap in the yoga universe, a connection to ancestry that had been lost. I set out to rescue a purist strand of the practice, stripping away everything that was allegorically Hindu, everything reminiscent of the 1960s hippie culture, everything influenced by American marketing, and everything tied to religion. I understood that the true value of my work, even on a spiritual level, is to serve this profound purpose in an artisanal way, helping individuals experience a reawakening, like turning on a light with a dimmer. Then, mind and body expand together, until they cease to be separate entities and become a single system.

All of this is connected to Buddhism. It aligns with the idea that there is no pain that does not originate in the mind, just as there is no bodily pain that can be dissipated without involving the mind.

People's lives are often marked by hip degeneration. No surgery can completely solve this issue. One cannot create the illusion that surgery corrects an entire history. It may address the immediate crisis that the history generated, but the story continues, potentially leading to further harmful, painful, or pathological consequences. In surgery, the most damaged tissue can be repaired or replaced, but the energy matrix that gave rise to the damage remains intact.

That's what yoga is about, the dissolution of the energy matrix that generates suffering. This is only possible when the mind stops its incessant thinking, allowing us to enter a place of deep self-knowledge.

When I began to grapple with the impact of the gunshot I experienced as a child and the joint and cartilage damage inside my hip, I felt as helpless as a dog hit by a car at the side of the road. I was in a cold sweat, trembling uncontrollably, with tears streaming down my face and experiencing excruciating pain.

But, within this investigative process, I was certain that I needed to uncover what was hidden. I kept revisiting that same position, moving through the middle of the pain, again and again and again until I discovered that I needed to go beyond the obvious sensations. And then, I learned to accept the pain, to welcome it, but never to identify with it.

Pain refers to something that is within you but does not belong to you. It is something that needs to be removed. If you attack it, it reacts. When you approach pain in a therapeutic process, with kindness, and infused with the right amount of self-care and self-love, it begins to dismantle the issues. It dissolves the problem.

It directs you to the place that yoga points us towards, the place of human potential.

That, is pure beauty.

Now, to return to Camila. How did she discover the unique potential of Kaiut Yoga? How did this discovery inspire her to mobilize others who would also play decisive roles in expanding the method throughout Rio Grande do Sul, starting from the Serra Gaúcha?

In addition to her practice and self-perception, Camila integrated her knowledge in natural health—such as Wilhelm Reich's organotherapy and Alexander Lowen's bioenergetics—with the content of Kaiut Yoga, all while continuing to question.

When I started Francisco's course in Curitiba, he had a reputation for being rude to people. He was known for not answering students' questions or responding in an unpleasant way. But I thought, "I leave my house in the countryside, leave my son, take a bus to the capital, then a plane, and from the airport in Curitiba it takes me another hour to get to the class. Am I supposed to stop asking questions? No!" If he was rude, it would hurt, but only my ego. So, I asked a lot of questions, and many times he didn't answer. It was a very cold, almost weird experience.

I never took it personally. I kept trying to understand why he was like that. I even campaigned with the other students to encourage them to ask questions because no one else was asking. There were yoga teachers, physiotherapists, and an orthopedic doctor, but no one asked. They said,

"Curitibanos—people born in Curitiba—are just cold like that."

I replied:

"That's ridiculous! You have many questions in your mind, yet you keep answering them with the knowledge you already have. But he's talking about something completely new. You won't understand it with the knowledge you already have. The guy is the creator of the method! You have to get into his head to understand. You must ask him!"

At the end of training, the class shifted their focus and entered a nebula of gossip. I didn't get into it.

"There is a man and there is a teacher. I relate to the teacher. The Francisco you're talking about is not the same as mine. I'm not going to get involved in this soap opera-like drama."

I wasn't going to lose my purpose.

Over time, he encouraged people to ask questions. To ask intelligent questions, that is. The personal turmoil only strengthened my connection with him and deepened our work together. When he returned, I admired his ability to navigate emotional storms and turn chaos into something positive.

Before my first class in Curitiba, the diplomatic atmosphere of the place caught my attention. There were no mantras, no incense, and no images. It was an environment that welcomed people of all religions. I realized that I would not be learning about chakras, which are always present in traditional yoga courses. I was fed up with that! What I wanted was to understand the students' pains. Not just the physical ones, but those that transcend the physical.

It was not easy to understand what Francisco proposed at first, but as he explained and presented his way of working with yoga, I became increasingly enthusiastic about what he had achieved. His approach combined neurosciences with natural therapies and the evolution of human movement. I had tried to intertwine all these elements before, but there was always a gap. Francisco managed to create this interconnection, adding a sense of grace to the process.

When we harmonize the body and the mind, generating a spontaneous meditative state, we come into contact with the unconditioned sphere of our being. This has a systemic effect, which is the charming proposal of the method. Francisco was truly incredible in connecting all these aspects without losing focus on the broader goal.

Francisco was incredibly effective in connecting all these elements, without placing an overwhelming focus on any element, like neuroscience or yoga. This balanced approach helped me understand what I was doing with yoga in the classroom. It served as a crucial guide for me in understanding health.

That was the definitive turning point for me. There was a significant gap between pain and the use of the body, and psychological and emotional pain. Francisco managed to integrate the best of everything, bringing yoga out of the dark.

A teacher from Porto Alegre called me, asking if I could teach a Kaiut class at her school. Out of respect for Francisco's work, I called him to ask if he would be willing to go and teach. He thought it was a cool idea, but the teacher specifically wanted me instead. Francisco authorized me, so I went.

That's where the desire to bring Francisco to Rio Grande was born. I remembered an earlier attempt by a girl from Curitiba and her husband, which hadn't worked out. I called him,

"Is there still that desire of yours to come to Rio Grande do Sul, work with the gaúchos, and bring your method here? Can we revisit this idea?"

He replied,

"It's actually a dream of mine to do this!"

"Then, my dream is your dream. I want and need to bring your work to my friends and the yoga teachers here. This method has the potential to revolutionize the history of yoga in Rio Grande do Sul. I don't mean to belittle anyone, because everyone here has a genuine motivation to help others. Bah! When you find a Ferrari, you don't want to drive a Volkswagen Beetle anymore, right?"

"Bah" is a very typical local gaúcho expression, meaning something akin to "wow!"

After that, I called Evelise from Caxias, who was taking a therapeutic yoga course in Garopaba, in the nearby state of Santa Catarina. I was very bold, I admit,

"Get out of there! This isn't even real therapeutic yoga. I've just discovered something much better. Come on, things are good. And bring your people along!"

Wherever Eve went, she brought a group of her students. I had my own network of contacts, including the people from the vibrant Lage de Pedra hotel and a very well-connected journalist who was also my student. She was a local correspondent for the *Correio do Povo* newspaper, the most respected print media outlet in our state, based in Porto Alegre. I think we ended up enrolling about 35 people in the workshop.

It was great because I already had experience promoting Iyengar teachers that I brought in. Despite their big names, usually just 17 to 20 participants would attend. From then on, everything became easier. The doors opened. I started bringing people to Francisco's workshops here in Gramado through the classes of the method I had been teaching in Porto Alegre, Caxias, Igrejinha, Farroupilha, and even Canela, paving the way for him.

And then, people who are now icons of the method, such as Luciana Costa from Porto Alegre, came to take the training course in Gramado. We managed to bring Francisco directly to Porto Alegre and later, with Eve, to Caxias do Sul. Things progressed from there. The teacher training course started at the end of 2017 with about 50 students enrolled, attracting people from all over Rio Grande do Sul to Gramado.

Sometime later, Ravi began organizing the events to give them more of a professional touch. I understood and was supportive, and I enjoyed collaborating with him too. When the pandemic hit and it became impossible to hold in-person workshops, they transitioned to online. I joined the sales team for the app they created. Our network in Rio Grande do Sul helped to sustain and grow the project.

When the possibility of in-person events returned, the idea of the Summit was born, a collaboration between Francisco and Ravi. Francisco invited me to take part as the connector, the person who brings everyone together, given my extensive involvement with the work.

So, who is Francisco for me?

He is an incredibly wonderful spiritual friend. Our relationship has never been affected by any psychological projection of needing a teacher or a father figure. When I met him, I was already well-resolved, having undergone therapy to address my relationships with men and with spirituality, due to a not very functional relationship with my father. This allowed me to collaborate with him without any anxiety about the male figure in front of me.

And he is a great teacher. A genius at what he does. Tireless in his pursuit of constantly improving his own creations. Always experimenting, testing new things. So, he's also a scientist. Very creative, incisive, and persistent, sometimes driving everyone around him crazy with his sense of urgency...

And, Kaiut Yoga?

It is the high tech of the high tech of yoga.

As we've just met Camila, the pivot of Francisco's journey in the gaúcho lands, we will next have the pleasure of meeting another two main figures in this journey, which is getting more and more exciting, as the method continue its expansion across its native lands.

16

On the Horizon, a Next Level

While we've just been in the Serra Gaúcha region with Camila and the growing Kaiut community, we need to delve deeper in getting to know this area—one that, interestingly, has had a connection to yoga even in its more distant past.

The Serra Gaúcha is a striking mountainous region that stands in stark contrast to the predominantly flat landscape of Rio Grande do Sul. In the realm of tourism, it is renowned for its carefully cultivated reputation, with its allure centered around the cities of Gramado and Caxias do Sul. Gramado, known for its rich German immigrant legacy, continues to exude strong Bavarian influences in its culture and architecture. Caxias do Sul, by contrast, showcases the heritage of Italian immigrants from the Veneto region. This Italian wave of immigration was instrumental in the establishment of the metalworking industry but more famously, significantly advanced viticulture in the area, which eventually gave rise to the National Grape Festival, "Festa da Uva". First held in 1931, this Festival has evolved into a major event, blending gastronomy, music, arts, and agro-industrial exhibitions. The 2022 event drew over 350,000 visitors during its 15-day biennial celebration, solidifying its role as a cultural highlight of the region. Italian immigration continues to shape the city, sometimes in unexpected ways, such as its connection to yoga and the introduction of Kaiut Yoga in the city.

Evelise Pisani, Eve, the granddaughter of Italian immigrants, recounts the arrival of yoga in the area:

My mother, Ivete Pisani, opened the first yoga school here in Caxias do Sul in 1978. It was a traditional yoga school, Yoga World Center. Today, at 88, she has retired from teaching but continues to practice as a student of the Kaiut Yoga method.

I began practicing yoga at the age of 16. Later, I went to Porto Alegre to pursue an undergraduate degree in psychology at the Pontifical Catholic University (Pontifícia Universidade Católica do Rio Grande do Sul (PUCRS)). After returning, I specialized in organizational psychology and worked for a metallurgical company. When I left, I worked as a clinical psychologist until 2001.

I've always practiced a lot of yoga, not just with my mother but with various other teachers as well. When my career as a psychologist began, I quickly realized that I could help my patients more effectively with yoga than with psychology alone. This realization motivated me to deepen my involvement with yoga, beyond just personal practice. I completed my teacher training and began collaborating with my mother at her school.

My focus was on hatha yoga. In 2015, Camila Moscarelli invited me to learn about Francisco's method. Attending his lecture in Gramado, I was shocked.

Francisco claimed that everything about the yoga we practiced was wrong. My initial reaction was to think he was crazy!

The next shock came during his class. I had always thought I was doing well in both practicing and teaching yoga. However, Francisco put me in certain positions and pointed out many things that were not right, which could potentially lead to problems in the future.

One of the things he showed me was that in the sukhasana position, sitting with my legs crossed, I appeared to bend forward gracefully. However, this masked underlying hip stiffness, as I was actually not moving much and was far from reaching the ground.

Another glaring issue he pointed out was that I had no movement in my neck. At 17, I had a car accident involving a frontal collision, which caused my right shoulder to reach my ear. Despite undergoing two surgeries to recover movement, I believed I had full neck mobility because I could perform various yoga positions. However, no other yoga teacher before Francisco noticed that I was compressing the vertebrae. Due to my injury, I should have avoided yoga positions where the weight fell on my head. My current challenge is still to move my neck, and with Francisco's method, I am now achieving a few centimeters [a little more than an inch] of movement.

I started to consider the possibility that Francisco's insights were accurate. Have you ever had the curiosity of realizing that your hips and spine don't move as they should? I noticed that many of the pains I was experiencing could be related to this. So, I decided to give it the benefit of the doubt and started testing his suggestions.

At first, when I heard him speaking, I wanted to run away. My initial thought was, "I'm not coming back here anymore!" However, I did return, but only to the familiar comfort of my usual yoga practice, where I didn't have to cope with the discomfort in my body or myself. Despite my initial resistance, I didn't give up. I began practicing and found a way to attend all of Francisco's workshops whenever he was in town. Eventually, I underwent his training and became a certified teacher.

In my practice, for a while, I would place my mat down for Hatha Yoga, occasionally trying a position or two from Francisco's method. Yet, I felt my body gravitating towards the experiences I had with Francisco more and more. Eventually, I began alternating between teaching Hatha Yoga and Kaiut Yoga at school. I soon realized that my approach was contradictory.

I could feel the benefits of Francisco's method in my own body. I saw tangible results in my students as well—those who came with pain, with serious hernia issues, or injuries began to feel better. They reported having bodies that were ready for life's activities, whether traveling or having fun. This inspired me to negotiate a license and change the school's name to Kaiut Yoga Caxias in 2022. From that point on, I committed to exclusively teaching Francisco's method.

To this day, some people ask me,

"Why did you do that? Your school is a school of tradition, the oldest still in operation in Caxias, and you chose to change?"

My response to them,

"I'm not changing anything. This isn't just a simple change of name or method. This is the evolution of yoga itself! It is a functional method aimed at ensuring well-being over the years. It represents a commitment to both physical and mental health. It's a loving approach to yoga, designed for everyone, because it honors and cares for the life story that is imprinted on your body."

This path on which I have placed myself is without return. Francisco once told me that the first time he saw me in a class, he thought, "I'm going to teach such a good class that this teacher will never let me go." And indeed, I haven't let go!

And now, looking back at all of Francisco's work, I'm reminded of what was once said about Iyengar. Before he died, Iyengar remarked that his work must not die with him. It should continue to evolve through his students. Within the timeline of yoga, Francisco is doing even more with his method.

Not only has he ensured that ancestral yoga stays alive, but he is pushing its boundaries even further.

While Eve brought her knowledge of psychology to her journey with the method, Luciana Costa—a pioneering teacher and owner of the first licensed school in Porto Alegre—brought her dual expertise as a doctor and pharmaceutical researcher.

Pain led me to yoga in 2010 and to Kaiut Yoga in 2016. My journey into yoga came many years after undergoing a very scientific, Cartesian classical medicine training at the Rio Grande do Sul Federal University in Porto Alegre. However, the doctor within me was already evolving, seeking not a return to some unachievable perfect state of health, but rather a reconnection with the natural ability of human cells to achieve balance, homeostasis. I had already come to understand this, and science supports it in many ways. The Kaiut method harnesses and delivers this inherent capacity for balance.

I was filled with chaos when I first came to yoga. After spending several years conducting clinical research on diabetes drugs and traveling the world constantly, I ran a company with partners providing services to the pharmaceutical industry. Eventually, I transitioned to working solely in my office. However, I was utterly normotic, teetering on the edge of psychosis, completely drained by ego, and a workaholic managing three cell phones, with no connection to myself. I was dying inside, at the age of 42, experiencing a complete ego rupture. On July 7, 2010, I disintegrated in a classic burnout. I became so disconnected that I even required psychiatric care at home.

A month later, I found myself in a yoga school. Despite having already completed a master's and doctorate in endocrinology, I began to study extensively, not only medicine and neurosciences but also philosophy, psychology, and the works of Freud, Jung, Socrates, Plato, and Nietzsche. Driven by anxiety and a need to relieve my pain, I came across a book by Deepak Chopra, *Perfect Health*, on Ayurvedic medicine. The subject captivated me. Like me, Chopra is an endocrinologist but based in the United States. His work helped me approach everything with an open mind.

I then treated myself with Ayurveda and pursued specialized training in this field with the renowned Brazilian doctor José Ruguê, who operates an Ayurvedic training center in Araguari, in the state of Minas Gerais.

By this time, I was growing frustrated with classical medicine as I continued to treat my chronic lower back pain, which had been flaring up since I was 24. My condition initially improved with yoga in the Iyengar tradition. However, I began overcompensating with my left shoulder through excessive weight training, which worsened my condition. This led to a highly rigid body and a left shoulder syndrome that caused weekly bouts of pain radiating to my neck, along with tingling in my face and hand. I pursued treatments with homeopathy, massage, chiropractic care, Ayurveda, and classical yoga. By then, I had already integrated Ayurveda into my clinical practice.

In 2016, I also began studying the practice of somatic experiencing, developed by Peter A. Levine. I realized there was an interesting path here and noticed that many people worldwide were discovering it as well. However, I soon recognized a blind spot: there was a need to integrate this new knowledge with yoga.

That's when I came across a Facebook or blog post with some exciting news. It mentioned something like "a man who practices yoga combines yoga with neuroscience and creates a method." I knew I had to learn more about it! However, I didn't want to travel. I had already spent a significant part of my life on the move and wanted to stay quieter in Porto Alegre. The news provided little information, but I knew that this man was in Curitiba.

A month later, I came across a copy of *Yoga Journal Brasil* with an advertisement on the back cover for Francisco's school in Batel, Curitiba. It felt like a sign. I asked the yoga school I was attending if they knew of Kaiut

Yoga. No one had heard of it, yet it was already making waves in the United States and Curitiba.

At the end of the year, I attended a new-age retreat in Canela. Camila Moscarelli was scheduled to teach yoga there. When I met her, she was holding a binder, like the ones used in FDA [the U.S. Food and Drug Administration] research for medicines, food, and medical products in the United States. The folder had an Americanized look with a large letter "K" on the cover.

I asked her what that was. She replied,

"I'm taking a training course with Francisco Kaiut in Curitiba."

"I can't believe it! I came to this retreat to learn about this course! Because I've been looking for this man!"

Camila then informed me that Francisco would soon be coming to Rio Grande do Sul and that she was gathering interest for a possible training course with him. I asked her to inform me in advance of his visits. However, the next three times he came, our schedules didn't align because I had other trips planned, including one to India.

Finally, on May 15, 2017, I was going to be in Porto Alegre when Francisco would be giving a lecture at a club near my office in the evening. The following day, there would be a class.

I spent the day excited by the idea that I would finally meet the man whose work I felt could significantly impact my practice. While studying Peter Levine's somatic experiencing, I had not yet fully grasped how to apply that knowledge practically in my office. However, I was confident that Francisco Kaiut's method had made significant advances along the same lines as Levine's.

I sat in the front row. There were only about 10 people. Francisco arrived somewhat shy, with a distinct Polish demeanor, holding a chimarrão—the typical gaúcho mate —in his hand.

My work in the office was already evolving. I was no longer just about being an endocrinologist treating diabetes. I was becoming increasingly interested in what the World Health Organization (WHO) would later term integrative health. This shift was transforming how I cared for both myself and others. I moved away from a paradigm of dependency on medication, expensive supplements, and practices that required numerous sessions. I had begun to adopt a more human-centered approach, viewing pain as a guide to restoring function and educating individuals about their own bodies.

I had seen in a lecture on somatic experiencing that Peter Levine reviewed the activation states of the autonomic nervous system, but this approach required the individual to be dependent on a therapist. In contrast, integrative health emphasizes empowering individuals to manage their own well-being without relying on external dependency.

I believed that a practice like yoga could offer this independence. During Francisco's lecture, my question was precisely about this topic: whether he was able to shift from the autonomic nervous system to the parasympathetic system through bodily practice.

Francisco's response, which I interpreted as positive, left me further enchanted with the method. The next day, I experienced it firsthand in his class. Although he was unaware of my shoulder pain, he guided me deeply into my body, helping me reach a place I never thought I could access. I finished that first class in meditation, feeling a profound state of presence due to the shift in my nervous system.

Camila was eager to learn more about me and my thoughts. I jokingly said,

"I want to stay here, meditating longer, without anyone else making noise at the end of class. Besides addressing my shoulder pain, the class validated the method for me. Perception of the body changes the frequency of the nervous system. I'm going to sign up for the training course!"

My intention was not to become a yoga teacher. I wanted to integrate the training into my professional practice as a doctor. However, in the fourth month of the course, while treating patients with diabetes, obesity, thyroid issues, arthrosis, and neuralgia in my office, I found myself teaching without even realizing it. I wanted to help, so I instructed my patients to sit on the floor and place their hands in certain positions. Before I knew it, I was teaching them how to do sukhasana.

At this stage, the girls from Caxias who were taking the course had already begun discussing opening schools for the method and obtaining licenses from Francisco. During a break at the café, one of them mentioned to me that no one from Porto Alegre had shown interest. I was initially reluctant. I didn't want to open a school. However, when another girl later said that someone needed to open a school in Porto Alegre, I found myself unexpectedly replying,

"I'll do it!"

In 2018, a month after completing my training, I opened the first Kaiut Yoga school in Porto Alegre, in the Auxiliadora neighborhood. In March 2022, I relocated the school to Moinhos de Vento, a prestigious neighborhood in the city. I brought on Ana Cláudia Costa (no relation to me) who was a former student and now a teacher of the method, along with a prosperous business person from the Porto Brasil travel agency, as a partner.

Nowadays, more than ten percent of our students are medical doctors, including rheumatologists, neurologists, pediatricians, and gynecologists. This is a clear sign of the growing openness of both local and academic medicine to integrative health.

Francisco is the visionary guy who recognized something straightforward: the cell's regenerative response to the constant stress imposed by Nature. This response occurs on physical, mental, and emotional levels. The Kaiut method serves as a precious and obvious tool, helping us reclaim what we've lost. Modern humans have forfeited the essential mobility functions of the human body, but this method restores various healthy bodily functions.

Kaiut Yoga, through focusing on joints and mobility, rescues the systemic process of cellular homeostasis, culminating in a state of spontaneous meditation. We are currently facing two pandemics: firstly, the inflammatory syndrome responsible for degenerative diseases, autoimmune conditions, cancer, hypertension, and diabetes, and secondly, the disconnection of individuals from themselves, manifesting as anxiety, psychosis, and other mental health issues. For all these ailments, there are lengthy lists of apparent remedies.

The method is the solution. It makes your mind clearer so you can choose what to eat to counter against the pharmaceutical and food industry that are next door, and that the method goes against. And it provides you with a body capable of evolving, expanding consciousness, so you can break free from antidepressants that dull your mind. It empowers you to navigate the challenges of making the best choices for your well-being.

The practice of the method is constantly evolving. It has evolved in Francisco, in me, and in all practitioners. It will guide us to new places because it is always moving forward. Francisco possesses an extraordinary intellect to observe the processes in Nature, within himself, and within us. He continuously updates the method with a solid scientific foundation.

You may have noticed that Luciana is situating the development of the method within the troubles and challenges of the broader context of the twenty-first century, such as those related to the pharmaceutical and food industries. These challenges are not isolated but are part of a larger, longstanding worldview—one that has, for a long time, upheld a homogeneous and rigid understanding of society. This limited perspective has perpetuated a simplistic portrayal of reality, shaping how we perceive and engage with the world around us.

At the heart of this worldview lies a paradigm—a mental framework that dictates our interpretations and responses to life. Paradigms act as filters, shaping our beliefs and assumptions—for instance, the belief that Nature exists solely for human exploitation. Such a mindset results in the disregard for Nature's cycles of renewal and regeneration. This mindset has led to unsustainable practices, such as year-round fishing; yet we later lament about the disappearance of species like the peacock bass, a prized ingredient in Amazonian cuisine, from our restaurant menus.

The predominant model of medicine and the way we address health issues stem from certain entrenched views that, over time, inevitably collapse and exhaust themselves. Such moments also spark necessary renewal where new perspectives and models can emerge, revitalizing society. Kaiut Yoga is such a revitalizing initiative—it offers a specific vision that contributes to the broader, proactive transformation of the world for the better.

In the field of health, figures like American chiropractor Joe Dispenza and pioneering epigenetic researcher Bruce Lipton also exemplify this renewal. Their work is intrinsically tied to the expansion of human consciousness, challenging outdated paradigms and enabling us to view both ourselves and the world through more enlightened lenses. These new approaches foster sustainable ways of living, replacing the ignorance and distorted values of the past with growing wisdom and awareness, guiding us towards a healthier and more conscious future.

Luciana:

This is how human beings evolve. Paradigms fall because, over time, they no longer make sense and create more imbalances. For example, sweeteners were once considered beneficial, but over time they've been linked to Alzheimer's and cancer. We have also turned to practices like bodybuilding, CrossFit, meditation, and yoga, but sometimes these have yielded dubious results.

Science has shown that if we didn't get sick, if the best-selling common medicine wasn't the antidepressant, and if we weren't dying from heart attacks, we wouldn't need to discuss paradigms that no longer serve us. What unbalances and disconnects us are the processes of making wrong choices.

A few years ago, we studied Ozempic, which the FDA approved as a diabetes drug in 2017. It didn't work as intended for diabetes. However, its side effect of making people nauseous and eventually losing weight led to its use as an obesity medication six years ago. Today, it's common for patients, even those from low-income backgrounds, to request prescriptions for this drug. People often want four boxes or more of the drug, and it's hard not to respond to their requests. However, you know that simply taking this medication won't solve their underlying problems.

Fortunately, there are others like Francisco and Luciana within the health field, trailblazers offering alternative paths to transformation. Art and science are evolving, delivering fresh insights, while philosophy and education continue to play vital roles in this ongoing shift. Many individuals are embracing change, and progress has occurred. But there is still a long way to go. And conflict with the powerful pharmaceutical and food industries is inevitable.

Francisco sees the roots of the dominant conservative health paradigm—particularly in the United States—and in nations under its cultural and economic influence—as an orchestrated act of population control.

Today, we live in an alarming situation where people are disempowered when it comes to their health. This is the result of fear marketing used by the medical system. We are told to seek specialized medical professionals for even the simplest issues and to consult a nutritionist before changing our diet. We're reminded not to miss our annual check-ups at prestigious hospitals like Einstein, Beneficência Portuguesa, or Sírio-Libanês in São Paulo. However, choosing a more expensive medical system might feel like validating your life, it doesn't necessarily mean you'll be healthier.

Everyone talks about the discoveries and advancements in medicine, but no one discusses what medicine has yet to uncover. No one educates individuals to understand the relationship between cause and consequence in their life choices, which deprives people of the desire to learn more about themselves. If you consult these little artificial intelligence robots about the negative impacts of hip surgery, they'll acknowledge their existence. But if you seek more information, they'll advise, "talk to your doctor." No search engine wants to risk engaging in a legal or judicial debate with the current medical system.

The message is clear: you're encouraged to not think for yourself. You need a medical professional. This dependency can lead to desperation. And often, you might hear, "there's nothing wrong with you. I think you'd better talk to a psychiatrist."

That's why, from the very beginning of developing the method, I understood I needed to create something different and independent, not just another medical solution. I recognized the necessity for a distinct language and approach, focused on student empowerment. It was about teaching students to make peace with what they feel, even when it's uncomfortable.

Nature wants to regenerate itself. But you may not want to feel this process. Sometimes, you may not be able to feel it temporarily. This raises important questions, in not feeling, in not going to these areas of discomfort, what are you protecting? Is not feeling protecting you or is it actually protecting the problem? Because pain has a *cunning nature. It can remain dormant for a long time, growing stronger. And then, by the time you realize it exists, it's already big and challenging to deal with.*

You can find the science that supports certain protocols or treatments for pain relief. However, there is often a lack of evidence to show that these improvements are sustainable in the long-term. Unfortunately, research indicating the ineffectiveness of certain treatments often doesn't reach the public or those suffering from pain. This selective dissemination of information can be misleading and harmful.

For instance, medications are typically deemed acceptable by scientific standards, but a closer look at their package inserts reveals significant risks and potential side effects. Similarly, supermarkets may sell bread containing chemicals that are banned in several other countries. This manipulation of scientific information raises serious concerns about the true motives behind these practices, which seem disconnected from genuine care for human well-being.

You might come across a survey or study that addresses your health concerns positively. But it is essential to ask: who financed this study? Because researchers can make their research can say whatever they want based on their intention. A well-known scandal from a few years ago exemplifies this issue. Research funded by Coca-Cola attempted to downplay the harmful effects of sugar in soft drinks. This example highlights the need for critical examination of research sources and potential biases.

Francisco is referring to a case investigated by *The New York Times* in 2015, which was also covered by the Brazilian business trade magazine *Exame* in 2023. The investigation revealed that

Coca-Cola sponsored scientific research to downplay the role of soft drinks in the increase of obesity and type 2 diabetes.

The article highlights other examples of questionable relationships between research institutions, including those affiliated with universities, and industry in the United States. These relationships often impose "truths" on public opinion that benefit businesses but harm individuals. Other classic examples include the tobacco industry, which for years funded studies that concealed the health risks of smoking, and the American Society for Nutrition, who conducted research in partnership with the fast-food chain McDonalds.

I have no inherent resistance to medicine or medical doctors. There are times when you need to see a doctor, and that's perfectly fine. I believe that doctors are valuable tools in your healthcare toolbox, but they shouldn't be the whole toolbox. Ultimately, you make your own choices. Your lifestyle, your freedom over your own life, and your degree of self-understanding are all crucial. That's why I developed this method to empower individuals. It fosters self-knowledge by encouraging you to listen to your body and understand the expanse of your life. Pain is the gateway in this process.

You might agree that this method has a noble purpose. It aims to empower individuals by fostering self-knowledge. One of the overarching themes in contemporary society is the conflict between emerging paradigms and the false realities imposed on us. These false realities condition, control, and shape our individual and collective existence.

A great example of narrative art that figuratively exposes this issue is the classic science fiction movie series, *The Matrix*. If you haven't watched it, I highly recommend doing so! The series suggests that our world operates like a computer program, complete with rules, codes, and algorithms that dictate how things function. This "Matrix" acts as the invisible framework of our perceived reality. The structure governs and controls our lives and society, manipulating and shaping our worldview, implanting beliefs into our minds that eventually become accepted as "truths."

Like all forms of power, the Matrix seeks to perpetuate itself. It detests the emergence of innovative perspectives that diverges from and opposes its intrinsic beliefs. Consequently, it works against the natural evolution of humanity and society, which is driven by the youthful energy that fosters transformation. Thus, the Matrix resists new worldviews that challenge its established order, seeing anything that challenges it as rebellious.

At this point in the narrative, as you have noted, Kaiut Yoga fits within the broader thematic field of health. This immediately stirs a sense of restlessness in my mind. And perhaps, like me, you are wondering: Is there a health Matrix ruling the world? What are Francisco's thoughts on this?

Absolutely. To understand this better, we need to revisit a specific story.

At the beginning of the twentieth century in the United States, during a period of extraordinary economic growth and the early success of capitalism, industry leaders had a visionary idea. They realized that by uniting as an economic group, they could expand their businesses and potentially achieve economic hegemony for no less than 100 years.

Brilliantly, these guys designed a plan to increase and sustain their profits into the next frontier. And what would that frontier be? The pharmaceutical industry. But how do you establish a powerful, dominant pharmaceutical industry? By organizing the field of medicine.

They began regulating medicine and standardizing it into a single practice model: the allopathic model, what we might otherwise refer to as "conventional" medicine. Their main strategic move was to radically change medical education by leveraging the massive power of money in universities, teaching, and research. Publicly, the discourse was about raising the quality of medical practice and improving the health of the American population. However, their real intention was to exponentially increase profits and ensure the long-term profitability of the pharmaceutical industry through the sale of medications.

And what was their first big marketing campaign?

To discredit any practices rooted in natural remedies. All these practices were publicly undermined. The next campaign was the campaign of not feeling! The basic message being, "You don't have to feel pain anymore!"

Due to their economic power and the United States' emerging status as a global superpower, this model spread worldwide. These industry leaders succeeded in building their version of the Matrix, a system now imposed on humanity. In one Machiavellian stroke, they tarnished global health. Most importantly, and terribly, they managed to influence and guide human behavior for generations.

There is no one alive today on the planet who is not influenced by the fear of feeling... the fear of experiencing their own body...

and taking responsibility for their life. It's absolutely surreal because this was all orchestrated. There was a thought, a plan, and its implementation. This plan still guides science and research today. It fosters separation and disconnection, continually sowing fear. Always fear.

Suppose you want to delve into the historical origins of this real-life Matrix. In that case, you'll find scattered documents that weave together a compelling narrative where the financial ambitions of major industrial tycoons intersect with the political objectives of a burgeoning nation striving to assert itself as a modern economic empire. Within this story, you'll uncover a blend of actions—some defensible and even partially beneficial to society—layered with half-truths and ulterior motives. Like life itself, this narrative isn't a clear stream of crystal waters but a murky swamp from which the lotus flower of progress may emerge.

In all cases, behind the intentions—whether they are bad or not so bad—you can identify the values, principles, and worldviews that shaped this Matrix. Like it or not, it is a powerful component of the global village our world has become. For better or worse, it shapes much of how we think about ourselves.

The key players in the creation of this matrix are revealed in independent research and the book, *Rockefeller Medicine Men: Medicine and Capitalism in America*, by E. Richard Brown, a professor at the University of California's School of Public Health. Brown's book reads like a politically charged drama fitting for the plot of a Hollywood movie. Central to this story is John D. Rockefeller Senior, often referred to as the "founder of disease medicine."

At the dawn of the twentieth century, Rockefeller, an oil tycoon and one of the richest men in the world, foresaw vast opportunities in the emerging petrochemical industry. Building on the success of oil-based products like plastic, he recognized the pharmaceutical industry's potential to produce medicines and related accessories, such as packaging, from petrochemicals.

In addition to his business ventures, Rockefeller became a prominent philanthropist. He established the Rockefeller Foundation, a vehicle that not only bolstered his business interests in the political sphere but also allowed him to shape public health, education, and scientific research. He also established the first biomedical research center in the United States—today known as Rockefeller University, which has employed at least 26 Nobel Prize winners over the years. This development was motivated in part by the tragic loss of his grandson to scarlet fever.

He also collaborated with steel magnate Andrew Carnegie, who was intriguingly his rival in the race to become the wealthiest man in America. Like Rockefeller, Carnegie was a large-scale philanthropist with a focus on education. Together, they embarked on an ambitious project aimed at "modernizing" medical education.

They commissioned an extensive survey to assess the state of medical education in the country and lobbied the government to adopt the allopathic model proposed by the research report. They financed the creation of the first public health courses in universities across the United States, Canada, and England, and economically supported the modernization of medical education at prestigious institutions such as Johns Hopkins, Yale, and Vanderbilt. Additionally, they worked to discredit then-prevalent medical therapies like homeopathy and chiropractic.

Furthermore, the Rockefeller group purchased a stake in the German chemical company I.G. Farben, which was a giant in the industry at the time and financed eugenic research in Nazi Germany. They also sought to establish their medical model in China by opening a university in Beijing.

How successful was their plan?

According to Brown's research, of the 166 medical schools in the United States at the project's outset, only 76 remained after 15 years. This consolidation was driven by the imposition of a standardized curriculum and the dominance of the allopathic model. This process was supported by the American Medical Association (AMA), which received financial backing from Rockefeller and Carnegie's philanthropic organizations.

The book's introduction further reveals the true significance of their plans. Brown's analysis reveals that these changes weren't solely aimed at improving public health. Instead, they reflected a deliberate manipulation of social and political processes by a medical elite working in tandem with immense corporate wealth. The result was a system of medicine designed more to serve economic and hegemonic interests than to address humanitarian needs. A diverse and eclectic variety of curative modalities available to the American public were eradicated in favor of a single style of medicine that would become the predominant form in the Western world and a major force in global medical culture in the twentieth century.

If you're thinking this is a somewhat heavy, even scary story, you're not alone.

But you know what?

In the first film of the *Matrix* series, the protagonist, Neo, faces the challenge of choosing between a red pill and a blue pill.

Choosing the blue pill leaves one trapped in the illusion, while choosing the red pill opens one's perception to a reality that transcends the Matrix, revealing the organic and vital truth beyond the pathological bubble.

Kaiut Yoga naturally developed by choosing the red pill. And, as a student, the method is also like choosing the red pill. This original organic vitality has led to remarkable and unexpected effectiveness in areas of health that few could have envisioned. For instance, Kaiut Yoga has become a significant therapeutic resource for managing debilitating conditions like multiple sclerosis (MS).

To truly grasp how Kaiut Yoga impacts MS, it's best to hear directly from someone who has experienced its profound benefits firsthand.

So, let's continue forward into a sensitive and deeply moving story that awaits you.

17

Another Prism of Real Magic

Katie Gargiulo is a resident of El Dorado Hills, a quiet town of just over 50,000 people in California, 96 miles (155 kms) northeast of San Francisco. She worked for many years as a municipal civil servant in nearby Folsom. It was in Folsom that Francisco and the method came into her life in a perplexing way.

I went to class on Thursday night, not knowing much about what to expect. I didn't even know how to spell the name Kaiut. I had never seen a picture of Francisco. I went because my yoga teacher at the Leap Yoga studio, where I went once a week, was a little disappointed that I couldn't do many of the positions. She mentioned there would be a visiting teacher she had heard about, but she had no idea who he was. Even so, she thought I should go.

By this time, I thought I should try anything that came my way. My life as a horse rider, horse trainer, and dog trainer, along with my love for the outdoors and nature photography, had been significantly reduced. My world then became the wheelchair and being basically indoors.

The first impression I get is when I arrive at the parking lot—it was full. I thought, "Okay, that's a promising impression."

I arrived in my motorized wheelchair, which weighs around 425 pounds [193 kgs] and is made entirely of metal. A yoga studio is a place where people like to walk around, hug each other, and go barefoot. That's why I pay close attention to people's feet. Once I'm inside, I look around, searching for a spot where I can be part of the group, more or less, without getting in anyone's way. Then, I don't think about anything else. I just notice, "wow, there are so many people here!"

And then Francisco walks into the room. He crosses the space and comes straight to my corner. Unlike anyone else who talks to me, he casually kneels, as if he's been doing it all along. He crouches and says,

"May I ask you what put you in a wheelchair?"

He is not socially performing and sounds genuinely interested. I deduce that he is the teacher, from what I had observed there at the time. And then I reply, kind of apologizing,

"Oh, you know, I have MS. Multiple sclerosis."

Then, he just looks at me and says,

"Wonderful!"

Then I think, "this guy is crazy! Maybe he has never heard of MS. He doesn't know what happens! But he is here, between me and the door, upfront. And now, what do I do?"

At that point, he pushes me into the center of the room! If someone had asked me if they could do that, I might have let them, but he doesn't ask. He doesn't ask if he can!

The class simply begins. He spends at least a third of the time teaching next to my wheelchair in a room full of people practicing on yoga mats. I do some arm raises and neck rotations, the exercises within my ability.

My mother was a teacher, my uncle was too, and my father was, in a way, one as well. I've seen many teachers. And then I realize, "this guy is beyond everyone. Teaching is his gift and his passion, and he is wonderful."

When he finishes, he asks me,

"Can you come back?"

I say no that there is no vacancy, and the course is complete. But then he clarifies, asking if I can come back in six months, when he is back in the city. He looks me in the eyes and says,

"I can teach you how to move. The things you are doing to accommodate your illness are causing more harm than the illness itself. Come back. I can help."

He doesn't say it won't hurt. He doesn't say it's going to be easy. He doesn't say he can make me walk again. What he says is just that he can help me move.

And that was impressive. I had assumed my job was to minimize the effects of the disease on my life, but I had no idea how to do that. The things I had tried hadn't always worked well. In therapy, I was told the most important thing was to never get up, never move away from the wheelchair, never stand up without holding on to something, and never put myself at risk. Don't bend over, and don't take anything from the chair.

That's just the way it was. It seemed right at the time. But I didn't realize that therapy didn't consider any kind of progress. My goal was to go back to work as a legal analyst in the legal field for the city of Folsom because I needed insurance. So, for two years, I did nothing but sit in this wheelchair. I never got up. I lost every pound of muscle tone I had and gained a ton of weight.

Katie pauses briefly. Then, without warning, leaps to the distant past, to where and when it all began.

One night in 2013, I went to sleep. Everything was fine. I was 55 years old. The next morning, I woke up paralyzed.

It took doctors about eight days to figure out what it was. They admitted me to the neurological ward but couldn't understand why it had happened so suddenly. They first thought it could be Guillain-Barré Syndrome, but I said, "no, no, no!" They then began eliminating the things that could be. Eventually, they decided to do an MRI [Magnetic Resonance Imaging] of the brain, with contrast.

And then, the worst neurologist you can imagine just walked into my room, didn't look me in the eye,

"Well, we've come to the diagnosis that you have MS. And, in my opinion, because of your age, you will progress very quickly. You'd better come to terms with the fact that you're probably going to go blind because the optic nerve is particularly sensitive."

And then,

"Is there anything I can do for you?"

He broke the news as if he were saying something like, "It's raining outside. Oh, and maybe you'd better bring an umbrella and, oh, drive carefully, the streets are wet." All I was thinking was, "What?! What?! *Anything you can do?* Yes, get out of here! Go!"

Ah, the (stereo)typical medical sensitivity and the level of skill in human relations among doctors, which is common in American hospitals…

Fortunately for Katie, the hospital where she was admitted introduced a new type of professional to the patient care process. Their role was a blend of psychologist, confidant, counselor, general therapy advisor, and a crucial link between the patient, administration, insurance services, and the medical team. This designated professional—an absolute jewel of a person, she says— was the man who helped her out of the terrifying abyss where she found herself. He sat with her in the room, spoke serenely for an hour, and then launched a lifebuoy,

"You are a warrior. I don't want you to give up. We have a rehabilitation service outside of here, an intensive training camp. I'll talk to the insurance. If they authorize it, I want you to go. You might not like it, but I want you to go."

Katie would do anything to get out of the hospital. And she did. Six weeks of exceedingly difficult training to learn to move forward with her new life, confined to a dysfunctional body. It was a life, she says, in which the disease had shattered her self-identity into small pieces and thrown it in the trash. Katie couldn't ride horses anymore, which she loved to do, couldn't have sex anymore, and couldn't stray too far from a bathroom.

And then came the return to work, two years of precarious performance that turned out to be unsustainable, until she accepted early retirement. She spent four months at home doing absolutely nothing until her brain started working a little better again, and a friend, her former boss, convinced her to try yoga. Then came Francisco, over four years since the diagnosis. That first class with Francisco was on January 18, 2018, and the second was in July that same year, when he returned to Folsom.

He arrives. He doesn't teach me how to get out of the wheelchair. Francisco just says:

"I want you to go down to the mat."

Okay. I wonder how I'm going to do this. Let's see. There's no other way but to fall straight because I'm not sure I can turn my body to get out. So, I put the bolster under me, slide, and fall. And I get to the ground.

So, I see that something is possible. Progress is possible. I sign up for the courses and workshops that will come. Taking classes with him directly every day would be nice, but it's impossible. He will come to our little town every six months, mainly because he is traveling and teaching worldwide—in Holland, Canada, and, of course, Brazil.

It's tough to travel by plane in the United States with a motorized wheelchair that is just less than two feet [55cm] wide. The chairs often get damaged in transport and return unusable. Traveling to Curitiba is out of the question, and it's too far to drive to Toronto. It won't happen that he can be here with us as much as we would like.

Then he tells me:

"Do yoga regularly. But don't practice at home. You're not ready. Come to the studio here in Folsom. Take classes with one of my teachers. When I come back, join my classes. These classes of mine are like a visit to the dentist. You come to floss your teeth."

I love what he says. From that moment, I enter a steady progression.

When he later talks about a teacher training course at the Leap studio, I get excited. It would be practically in my backyard, just 15 or 20 minutes from home. I really want to participate, but I'm unsure if I can. I worry it might be too much for me or that I might hinder others in the classroom. So, I decide to leave the decision to the teacher. I ask one of the girls at the studio to inquire on my behalf. Francisco's response is typical,

"If she thinks she's ready, she's ready!"

"Thanks! That's a major help! Okay, I'm going to dive deep. I'll do it!"

I know it won't be easy. The course is intensive, with each class lasting a full day. In the past few years, I haven't done any consistent activity all day for eight consecutive days, except breathing. I know I'll be exhausted by the end of each class. But if there's one thing I've learned in therapy that's helpful for all of us with disabilities, it's that you can work on long-term goals. You can define where you want to be in X amount of time and then create a reverse schedule.

Happy, I write an article, The Kaiut Movement, sharing my experiences so far and announcing that I will be taking the teacher's course. I thank the teachers at the studio—Iwona, Molly, Butch, Stacy, Cindy, Michéal—and the entire Leap community. It is a moving text. I expected it would only be published on the studio's blog, but they send it to Francisco in Brazil as well.

When he arrives for the course, the first thing he tells me is,

"I loved your post! You wrote from the heart. I think you're loving my method."

"No, Francisco. I don't love your method; your method is changing my life!"

He's not really an emotional guy, it's as simple as that. So, he just says,

"Okay, I'm going to start my class."

And Francisco moves away.

From that point, he starts challenging me every minute, in every class, every day.

I love the forward folding position. Whether using the chair or using the wall, supporting my back, and then bending my body forward. I have super short legs but relatively normal arms. It looks cool, and I feel cool. Then I just collapse, and go back up, leaning against the wall and pushing myself up with my hands.

Then he approaches, and puts the microphone aside:

"Can you stand up without using your hands?"

I look at him, incredulous:

"Oh, I shouldn't do that."

"In my class, try what I suggest. Try it! Let me tell you something first. You're on a yoga mat in this room, and I'm right here. So what if you fall? What do you think will happen? You won't get hurt."

"Oh... okay..."

I then press off my legs a little bit. And raise my torso. And it is then that I hear Francisco use an expletive for the first time,

"This is fantastically badass!"

Then, on the last day, he teaches the entire class of 75 or 80 or so students from the back the gym, where I am situated. He makes me stand up. I am facing the wall, barely touching it, supporting myself the tips of my fingers. A portion of the class is sitting right next to me, ready to assist in case I pass out, can't handle it, or need help sitting back down. He doesn't look at me or give any specific tips. He's sitting, calling people by their names, and a good part of the class doesn't see me. But I've never felt so secure in my life.

Then he says:

"Guys, I know you've been working hard, but I want everyone to turn here now. Look here."

They turn around. And they see me. Then, there is a tremendous spontaneous applause. I break down crying. I can only say:

"Okay, I need to sit down now."

And he simply says:

"Okay, okay, fine. Now we can leave."

A new pause, a sigh.

I'm not someone who's easily dazzled. I'm skeptical by nature. I have a degree in Law. Though I'm hopelessly romantic, I am also deeply analytical. The reason I wanted to take the teachers' course was to understand the science behind it. I received a wealth of information, where it comes from, the history of the method, why it works, and much more. Once I knew all this, I was like, oh, of course, that's it.

With this attitude, Katie attends her second in-person teacher training course. Late January, early February 2020, when the dark clouds of the COVID-19 pandemic are slowly forming around the world.

Francisco knows that I've been practicing yoga diligently. He says,

"Very well, we have crossed a threshold. Now, I want you to do more standing work. I want you to free yourself a little more from the chair."

Once again, there are about 80 students in the room. He knows that some postures tire me, and I'm unsure if I should attempt them. At times, he insists, other times, he doesn't. Okay, I understand he's far ahead of me on this path. I accept whatever he says, whatever it is.

This is hard work! It's not a birthday party!

One day, Francisco tells me he knows I'm working hard, perhaps harder than anyone else in the room, because my response system doesn't work the same way as others'. On top of that, I have the aggravating factor of a knee injury. I've had four surgeries on my right knee as a result of a horse training accident. There's probably a lot of scar tissue, making it difficult to bend. The doctors told me, 'You have to be very careful.' It wasn't until Kaiut Yoga that I realized all I had been doing was supporting the knee injury, not the knee itself. So, while I can't do some of the postures, just trying them is amazing.

In this course, there's another person with a physical disability, Dave. Also present are Ravi—whom I am seeing for the first time—and his American friend, Jackson. Both follow Dave closely, paying a lot of attention, and they are Francisco's assistants. While all Dave can do initially is put his legs up against the wall, one day he walks away differently than he did before. He is changed— his face is relaxed, and his shoulders are less tense—because he worked on fear, pain, and his physical body. He comes to exchange experiences with me, as we obviously share a physical disability. Enthusiastically, he says,

"This is magic!"

But I correct him,

"It's magical, Dave, but it's the method."

Progress is undeniable, but life rarely moves in a straight line.

Then, the first major crisis of my illness occurred since starting practice. I lose all ability to stand. My left hand becomes useless, presumably because I drive with my right hand. I can move it, but I can't feel it. It's no longer safe for me to go down to the mat. I stop practicing.

After a long time, I send a message to Francisco via Telegram. I don't want to bother him or flood his Telegram or voice mail with messages. After all, he has what, like 10,000 students from a million countries to care for? It's my illness, and it's predictable, it happens. It's not fair to burden him with this, and poor me…

But then I get over it. Number one, because he cares about his students. Number two, he has the answers. In fact, what I have for him is a question.

"I can't get to the mat anymore. I'm trying to do the exercises in bed."

"How do you get to the shower?"

"I have a transfer board."

"Then go to Amazon and buy a massage table. Place the table at the height of the wheelchair. Use the transfer board to get onto the table. Place your legs up against the wall, it will be better for your back. Do the poses you can on the table. And regarding your left hand, review my video about hands on the teachers' platform."

I go back to practicing. It makes my third teacher training possible. And it changes my life.

When I say that he changed my life, I don't mean anything mystical or religious. It doesn't mean that I changed my hair color or lost weight. It means that my entire life has transformed because of his teachings. These are life lessons that have impacted my dog training, my relationships with people, everything. When I meet strangers, I don't back down anymore. People often approach me and ask what happened. Instead of seeing it as an intrusion, I now say, "Hi, I have MS."

This is the magic of this method and what it has brought to my life.

In classes, the magic is for everyone. There are emotional and physical reactions, exhaustion, breakthroughs, and incredible joy. It's absolutely amazing! The magic lies in the fact that everyone feels the class is tailored for them. Each person feels seen and cared for. No one goes without being called by name, receiving individualized attention, or personalized instruction. "How do you feel? ...I want a peak of intensity in those hips right now. ...Can you give a little more with your right ankle?" We are all having the best experiences.

And then COVID-19 hits. However, Francisco continues the course online. Although the video quality of the initial broadcasts in a Facebook live group is horrible, he is with us daily for the first 35 classes. Later, I also have classes with Ravi. This leads me to start practicing yoga every day.

This is a giant step in my transformation. I see the pandemic as a tool that opens opportunities for me, rather than a limitation due to the mandatory restrictions. I receive my certificate as a Kaiut Yoga teacher and start teaching— online.

People see me in a wheelchair and ask,

"But do you teach yoga?"

"Yes, I teach!"

When Francisco comes back to the United States for the first time after the pandemic for a special event in Boulder, I was determined to go. Even though it meant travelling interstate. Not even a firearm would have stopped me from going.

My husband was very worried. However, a friend of mine, a student, agrees to accompany me and push my wheelchair. This time, I use a manual wheelchair so I can get on the plane. The event it in a huge venue and attracted people from around the U.S. and from overseas. We've barely emerged from the threat of the pandemic, and yet here we are, hugging and crying, overwhelmed with emotion.

Then, at the entrance, I don't hear anything, but I feel someone touching my shoulders. You know who he is. I swear I won't cry, but I do. He says,

"Katie, what kind of wheelchair is this you brought? Where is your motorized super chair?"

"It's at home, safe, protected from planes..."

"You come all the way from California and bring this crap into my classroom!?"

"Oh, my God, no, no, no!"

I get ahead of myself. My sturdy motorized wheelchair would have been useful in getting to a standing position. I knew that this time he would give me the exercise of standing on the wedge and lifting myself, leaning on the wall. I suggest that I try to get up without the support of my hands, without anything. I say,

"Why don't we try? The worst that can happen is that I fall..."

He laughs and walks away, leaving the decision up to me. For the first time, I get up without any support, in the center of the room!

Katie began her career as an certified Kaiut Yoga teacher, working online through the Zoom platform, initially offering lessons one-on-one. When she believed she could also teach in-person classes, Katie imagined she could accommodate four students at a time. Without a location to hold these classes, she turned to her friends at Leap Yoga Studio to teach from their space.

Not only did they give her a space and time to teach from but also gave Katie the gift of five additional students. In her first in-person class had nine students.

And now you might be curious to know: what was the most important lesson from Francisco's teachings that she remembered when starting her in-person classes?

He's one hundred and ten percent right all along. He says that when you teach, you must not think about you. Think about the student. When your focus changes in this way, you see much more and can give much more to the student.

He emphasizes the importance of a deep commitment to the student—one grounded in connection, partnership, and genuine care. But for me, the only way to honor that commitment fully is through honesty. I tell my students,

"This is who I am, and this is what I've been through."

There may even come a day when I have to say during class,

"Today, I can't."

It's one of the few things that makes me a little frustrated with my situation.

But Francisco taught me not to throw myself into the pit of despair. I had to go through that kind of grief, the process of feeling like the universe hates me and that I didn't work hard enough. But I came out emotionally intact, spiritually intact.

There are people who ask me, "why aren't you depressed?"

Why should I carry depression with me?

He taught me something else. I told him that the rehabilitation staff had advised me to wake up every day and assess what wasn't working before getting out of bed. Here's Francisco's reaction,

"But why would you start your day doing something ridiculous like that? No! What you need to ask is something else: 'am I relaxed? Do I feel good? What is my body telling me? Is there anything that feels stronger today?'"

It's not about looking for the worst or creating a false sense of positivity but rather accepting the state of things, information without judgment.

One day, a new student, the husband of one of the Leap instructors, attends class. I put him in sukhasana and ask him to extend his arms. Then I notice that he is rocking his body back and forth, resembling someone with Parkinson's disease. I don't say anything. Instead, I simply bring him another bolster.

"This is not about effort or posture. It's relaxation. Just place your hands on the bolster. You don't need to stretch to the ground. Just relax in the position."

The words flow out of my mouth. As I speak, he stops shaking his body.

I explain to the student's wife, a traditional yoga teacher that is a mental pattern.

"You see students achieving beautiful results. These results don't have to be as spectacular as Dave's, who was able to leave the class walking steadily. It could be a student experiencing his first 30 seconds of peace in his system after a car accident."

This is success. The magic is in the method and the person behind it. It's a reproducible magic. I feel very privileged to have learned directly from Francisco and the people he taught. It's phenomenal!

Do you remember the scene from the classic movie *The Wizard of Oz* when the heroine, Dorothy, and her dog, Toto, land in the Land of Oz? Doesn't she open the door and the film changes from black and white to color?

That's exactly what Francisco did with the method.

"Look inside. You can get there."

"Really?"

"Really!"

And that's what happened.

She understands that Francisco dislikes the connotation of magic, as it can evoke notions of fantasy or illusion. However, Katie insists on interpreting the "magical" quality she attributes to the method within a natural context. Having heard Katie's experience, not we can return to Francisco, and his views on the function of the method, as well as its limitations, in cases of severe, chronic illnesses.

Multiple sclerosis is indeed a profoundly impactful disease, and it's common for individuals to associate nearly every bodily discomfort they have with the disease's progression. This association naturally amplifies their tension however, due to the inherent insecurity and fear it brings. For example, when the shoulder hurts, there is fear of a new crisis. When the hip hurts, fear arises, compounding the emotional toll of the disease.

My experience with multiple sclerosis is more extensive in the United States than in Brazil. One thing I've noticed is that much of my students' suffering does not stem directly from the disease itself.

When Katie first arrived in a wheelchair for class, I made sure she felt comfortable. I managed to move her away from a place of defense and fear, integrating her into the collective in a very inclusive way. From that point on, we developed a fantastic relationship.

I always tell her that we will address what has happened, but we must also prepare for likely future crises. Each new crisis will be a new discovery, and any potential losses will become the reason why we practice.

You can't confront a disease of this magnitude and create the illusion that we will directly impact the disease. No. Instead, we will focus on affecting the nervous system, regulating it. If this regulation has a positive effect on the disease, Nature will take care of the rest.

Her biggest discomforts were related to her knees, due to the wheelchair and previous knee issues. Even without having control of her legs initially, she ended up doing exercises while standing, outside the chair, reconnecting with her nervous system in profound ways. This process dispelled many physical discomforts that, while not caused by the disease itself, were mistakenly associated with it. Today, in my work with others who have multiple sclerosis, the approach remains the same: distinguish what is directly caused by the disease from what I call unnecessary suffering. It's essential to identify where the disease ends and where tension, emotional trauma, or other unrelated issues begin—often rooted in past experiences rather than the condition itself.

I have worked with some students who have Parkinson's disease. These students typically present with muscle stiffness, which is one of the main causes of discomfort and loss of physical power and vitality. When they commit to a long-term yoga practice, I've observed significant reductions in this rigidity.

The key to managing such conditions is embracing the disease with compassion while maintaining a clinical perspective. This allows us to recognize that much of the day-to-day suffering typically considered inherent to the disease may not actually be caused by it.

Individuals with complex conditions, especially those affecting the nervous system, tend to be highly focused and consistent students. This dedication enables them to explore their bodies in detail—joint by joint, cell by cell—identifying areas that may be underused or neglected, regardless of the disease. Through this practice, we see transformative improvements in their quality of life.

And when a student who already practices develop the disease, consistency becomes even more crucial. The presence of a condition is never an excuse to stop caring for oneself. Life continues, bringing challenges like falls, broken bones, or accidents—not because someone caused them, but because they are part of living. You don't practice despite the pain; you practice because of it. You don't practice despite the disease; you practice because of it.

I have an American student here with me in São Paulo right now. We're in the midst of a week of in-person work. She traveled from the United States for this. Years ago, she experienced hip pain. During a consult, I explained that it was not a hip problem, but rather hip pain. However, being young and resistant, she decided to undergo surgery. Unfortunately, not only did the procedure fail to improve her condition, but it also made things worse.

I took a trip back in time with her, searching for the thread to uncover both the biomechanical and emotional sources of her nervous system overload, and how these contributed to other issues. She was shocked to realize that she had spent several years trying to protect her hip with various methods that only worsened the situation.

When considering pain, it's important to understand that it is neither purely mechanical nor entirely Cartesian; it is fluid, dynamic, and systemic. Pain can be a movement, a signal. However, people often identify with their pain, believing it to be an intrinsic part of them. But pain doesn't belong to anyone—it simply exists, arising from a cause. Over time, avoiding pain only allows its complexity to grow.

For students with conditions like multiple sclerosis or Parkinson's, yoga provides a powerful opportunity to explore their nervous systems deeply. The practice fosters self-knowledge and helps separate the disease itself from the emotional, physical, and psychological burdens it may carry. By doing so, students can acknowledge the existence of the disease and accept the future unpredictability it entails. However, they can also come to understand that it doesn't need to dominate their daily lives.

Every disease begins as a pattern within the nervous system, long before it manifests physically. That's why we practice when we feel well—so we are prepared for the times we don't. And when don't feel well, we practice precisely because we aren't well.

Another student I had also attributed her specific issue to multiple sclerosis. I suggested it might instead be related to her spine. She resisted this idea, so I encouraged her to consult a doctor. After thorough investigations, it turned out not to be multiple sclerosis. Later, when she experienced a shoulder crisis, she again believed it was related to her condition. Once more, it wasn't. Through biomechanical reorganization, we worked together to dismantle the idea that every pain or limitation was tied to her disease. This realization liberated her, helping her see how fears and insecurities had amplified imagined connections to the disease. She began to view her condition from a more detached and empowered perspective.

For me, there's no such thing as Ed having multiple sclerosis. For me, there is only Ed—a person who needs care and education from a perspective of health and integrity. This approach is the best thing you can do for a student. When the student has no issues, he needs to learn to prepare, because at some point, the student might face challenges. When the student face challenges, the practice becomes a tool to navigate them. I try to instill the culture of practicing because of those challenges, not despite them.

One of my students, who had a severe rheumatic condition, shocked her doctor after regaining full mobility through yoga. Her arms, previously limited to shoulder height, could now extend above her head, and her medication needs had significantly decreased. Yet, instead of celebrating this improvement, her doctor saw it as a risk— an unfortunate reflection of a segment of medicine that views self-care and natural improvements as threatening.

I do not deny that an individual has multiple sclerosis, Parkinson's disease, or an autoimmune disorder. My view is not one of denial. I simply don't assume that the disease explains everything. I believe that if crank Nature's little machine, the disease maintains its place and size, especially considering this modern thing of so many diseases linked to the nervous system. Any disease that involves the nervous system must be treated by regulating the nervous system.

A matter of awakening awareness.

Medication does not teach individuals how to self-regulate. Instead, it often gives them the illusion of being in control. From a natural perspective, medications can actually make individuals more prone to generating negative, distorted, and sickening thoughts without them even realizing it.

What happens?

The human mind is powerful. When you start cultivating unhealthy thoughts, you eventually become incredibly good at it. You get so adept that you become highly skilled at generating anxious, tormented, and unhealthy thoughts. In essence, you develop a superpower: the ability to fry your own nervous system.

In our current social climate, the regular regulation of the nervous system is more important than eating. All known diseases, and those yet to emerge, are linked to the nervous system. The autonomic nervous system even regulates our metabolic health. You can eat healthy foods like arugula, but if you're operating from a stress pattern, it can still lead to high glycemic responses. There is no ideal diet if the nervous system is not in balance. What you eat will be distorted by anxious thinking and habits that undermine your internal health.

There was another student with a hip problem who initially thought her issue was due to being overweight. Anxious, she began engaging in a lot of physical activity. However, if one is anxious and tries to manage it through exercise alone, it can backfire. Physical activity is beneficial but using it to compensate for anxiety can be a ticking time bomb. Eventually, it will explode, because while the mind may become more anxious every day, the body cannot cope with an increasing exercise load indefinitely. There needs to be a balance. Just like a teeter-totter, if one end goes up, the other must go down. True equilibrium requires both ends to find balance.

I asked this student why she engaged in so much physical activity.

"Why do you spend two hours a day, pedaling on a stationary bike at the gym?"

"Because I love spinning."

Every anxious person says they love spinning. But they don't really love it, they love the feeling of being able to eat more and enjoy the sensation of exhaustion. However, at night, they don't sleep well, they sleep exhausted.

For some people with a moderate level of anxiety, this approach might temporarily work. But for the vast majority, the body reaches its limit first. This was the case with this student. Eventually, the accumulated anxiety overwhelms them. When the body can no longer serve as an outlet, and without proper self-education, the mind spirals out of control.

It is common to happen to people who run. People who destroy their hips and knees by running. They have not dealt with the nervous system throughout their lives. The knee is not the cause. The knee is the one that suffers the consequence of an indirect action. They think that the body will withstand this violence for the rest of their lives. They think that prostheses and surgeries will fix whatever issues have arisen; this is a very childish understanding of how the human body works.

I have encountered this issue frequently throughout my career, especially in the United States, where prostheses and surgical procedures are often performed incredibly early. At the first sign of discomfort, they rush to use the scalpel.

As a result, what I have seen is that each procedure is a blow to one's vitality in many ways. It's exceedingly rare to see a procedure without a significant negative impact, which often goes unnoticed. People have this desperate desire to avoid pain, lacking even the smallest inclination towards self-knowledge. They use their bodies as a disguise for their anxious minds and as a distraction from truly knowing themselves. It's alarming!

The prominent Matrix of sporting culture across the globe further fuels such attitudes and engagement with the body.

They cannot find peace because they drive their bodies to exhaustion, mistaking relentless activity for truly living. Yet, if you look closer, their vitality—their life force—is deeply depleted. Their sexual energy is drained, and what remains is an inability to achieve inner peace. What they truly need is therapy.

Often driven by poor self-image and a fixation on achieving a certain aesthetic, they engage in far more physical activity than is necessary for health—often much more than most people realize. Ironically, instead of promoting well-being, this excessive exercise leads to a loss of metabolic health. They age themselves on a chemical level. This happens because they don't want to look inward, unwilling to confront what lies within. In the process, they damage their hips, knees, ankles, and spines. They systematically breakdown.

All the while, they create the illusion that they are doing something wonderful. They fail to see how they are also being manipulated by industries eager to sell them sneakers, gear, and a fantasy of health. They confuse high-performance athletics with health, unaware that their lifestyle generates oxidative stress far beyond any actual health benefits. And what is the response from these industries? "No problem—let's throw medicine at it! Let's fuel the anxiety! And hey, let's buy more Nike!"

Running miles a day doesn't help anyone sleep well. It simply makes everyone sleep exhausted. Our culture glorifies overwork, excessive physical activity, and excess in every form. But where is the balance? At such a relentless pace, nothing can be seen clearly.

Even the so-called "pleasure" of running often has deeper roots within the nervous system. Many believe they run for enjoyment, but in reality, they run out of fear. Fear of becoming overweight like their parents. Fear of confronting insecurities and inner demons. They are not running toward health; they are running away from what scares them. It is a logic that is unhealthy and ultimately one that creates illness.

Consider the research used to justify prosthetic surgeries for joints. Much of it is ethically questionable, as it is often financed by the manufacturers of prostheses themselves. This is just one aspect of the broader commercialization of the disease industry. Running culture is a prime example: 94% of regular runners will eventually require hip or knee replacements. The more people push their bodies beyond their limits, the more prosthetics and surgeries are sold. The industry thrives, but individual health suffers. After all, peace of mind doesn't sell, nor does it lead people to become sick enough so these industries can profit from them. It's truly pathological to use one's body to the point of harming oneself in this way.

There is a psychological and spiritual aspect to this situation too. Why reach the point of such self-destruction and harm? What drives someone to this extreme absence of self-care?

The issue here is not with doctors or the procedures themselves. Modern medicine, in cases of trauma, can be miraculous. A hip replacement following a severe accident or a crushed femur is a blessing of medical innovation. Absolutely, go ahead and do it!

But what I question is the process that leads individuals to self-harm, and the medical discourse that perpetuates the illusion that such actions have no consequences—because, after all, "there are spare parts for the body."

This culture of excess also ignores the high rates of depression among former Olympic athletes who endure chronic pain and *disability. Instead of addressing these realities, we take rare exceptions as the rule. Yes, there may be an octogenarian who runs marathons, but for every one of these stories, there are hundreds who suffer from debilitating hip, knee, or spinal injuries. Modern competitive and corporate culture doesn't aim to nurture healthy elders. It demands unrelenting productivity until people are 60 or 70, leaving them to deal with the consequences alone afterward.*

The real battle in modern society is not David against Goliath, but the individual against illusion. The only way forward is to look inward, focusing on the body, on mindful movement, and on reconnecting with oneself. Only then can we break free from this destructive cycle.

Yes!

A strategic pause is needed now. The sound of silence. This is the depths of understanding at the heart of the Kaiut Yoga method, concerning the forces we are up against when it comes to our health.

As I mentioned at the start, in the mirror of this tale, you may have glimpsed parts of yourself, or those close to you, navigating this inner and outer minefield in search for true health and well-being.

Our journey it not finished yet—there are two more touching episodes and a little more to venture along. So, let's continue.

18

Movement... Transmutation

When the WHO declared COVID-19 a Public Health Emergency of International Concern in March 2020, the entire world suddenly faced an unprecedented situation of global paralysis.

Mandatory lockdowns confined populations to their homes, borders were sealed, and economic activity came to an abrupt halt across most sectors. Thousands of daily commercial flights, the lifeline of global mobility and trade, were suddenly grounded. Mass cultural and sporting events were canceled, and rising mortality rates across the globe cast a shadow of fear and uncertainty. These events could easily form the basis for a Hollywood dystopian thriller, perhaps aptly titled *The Day the Earth Stood Still*.

Everything seemed to change overnight, forcing individuals, institutions, and societies to adapt just to survive. The pandemic became a profound symbol of a larger dramatic shift in human history. A shift that, while triggered by the virus, was deeply rooted in the societal and environmental transformations unfolding since the 1960s and continuing into the 2020s and beyond. It was a turning point in every sense, impacting those who were thrust into change and those who saw the moment as an opportunity for reflection and transformation.

The concept of a turning point isn't new. Theoretical physicist Fritjof Capra captured it eloquently in his seminal 1982 book, *The Turning Point*. Capra warned of the dangers of an exhausted civilization caught in outdated paradigms— the very mechanisms of the Matrix that perpetuate chaos and disconnection. The book inspired the film *Mindwalk*, starring the renowned Liv Ullmann, which explored the emergence of new models of reality in science, art, and philosophy. Both the book and film envisioned a way forward—a rebuilding of society from the rubble of restlessness, with new seeds of hope and vitality planted in the human soul.

Where do Kaiut Yoga, Francisco, and each and every one of us fit into this picture?

Imagine a holographic environment where every part is interconnected, contributing to a unified whole. To navigate this landscape, we must embrace a systemic vision, a perspective that recognizes the interconnectedness of life and the possibilities of transformation. As we step into this kaleidoscope of challenges and opportunities, let's keep our feet firmly planted on the ground and our hearts calm and open. May this stage of the journey be as rewarding as it is illuminating.

When the pandemic struck, we took a huge hit, both financially and operationally. We were in a phase of expansion, with 40 team members including content producers, designers, marketing professionals, and journalists. Unfortunately, we had to reduce our workforce and lay off some valued team members. At the Batel school, which had about 600 students, we faced high operational costs, including rent and maintenance. Ultimately, we had to make the difficult decision to close the school. Licensed schools in Brazil had to close as well, facing severe and substantial problems, which resulted in considerable debt.

Since the divorce, Francisco had increasingly delegated business management and decision-making responsibilities to Ravi.

I never imagined thinking about expansion or opening schools, nor did I ever envision coordinating a business plan. It was never my dream or my vocation. When people said,
"This business of yours is not going to scale,"
I replied,
"So what?"
It's not in my nature to simply chase after money.

Fortunately, Ravi's entrepreneurial acumen and proactive leadership proved to be the perfect complement to Francisco's teaching. Their partnership became essential in navigating the challenges of the pandemic. Together, they found ways to sustain the vision of Kaiut Yoga through one of the most difficult periods in recent history. A testament to the resilience of their shared mission.

Much of what my father tried to do in partnership with others did not work out. It was frustrating because the same stories kept repeating themselves. Eventually, we decided that having partners wasn't the solution. From that point on, it was just the two of us, and that was it.

Using a brand licensing system, we had planned to expand from 25 to 35 accredited schools in 2020. We had already identified two possible expansion strategies: we could expand online or in-person. We chose to expand in-person, but the pandemic put an end to this plan.

We had to remodel everything, which is where we are now. However, we continue to work from our licensing model, which is not a franchise. Our idea is not to expand into a conventional type of business. That approach doesn't work for us.

Our model operates on an annual licensing fee, which grants the right to use the brand. Additionally, all teachers must engage in yearly professional development, remaining up to date with the method. All licensed schools are required to have at least one teacher certified by us, who must also remain up to date.

The hardest part is finding the right person for our business—someone who can effectively convey our vision without resorting to shortcuts or taking the easy way out.

Entering the North American market was super tricky at first, primarily due to currency differences. We earned in Brazilian Real but had to invest in U.S. dollars. Additionally, many yoga teachers in North America pursue teaching as a second or third career, rather than their primary occupation. Those who do focus on yoga as their main career tend to be more successful through commercial routes, selling the idea of physical activity in that of yoga, followed by the sale of clothes and accessories. Teaching regular classes to a consistent group of students is more complex than making money from events or workshops. This is the nature of the American commercial machine, and to enter this market, we must stay true to our values.

317

Therefore, now, our focus is more on solidifying our units [i.e. schools] in the United States rather than expanding. Right now, we have eight licensees in the U.S. and eight here in Brazil. We have achieved a structure where our revenue is evenly split, with fifty percent coming from the United States and fifty percent from Brazil. However, as a company, we are still relatively small. We don't yet have the financial strength needed to invest in the American market at the level required for significant expansion. What we are doing instead, is organizing dedicated events in California. In 2023, for the first time, I went there to teach.

In Europe, we have a base of teachers in Amsterdam. To create a European expansion model, I need to consider a unique approach for each country, as legislation varies significantly from one to another. I must also be cautious to avoid franchise legislation, since I don't have the capacity to deliver franchise services.

The current challenge is expanding by adding new units while grappling with the tough administrative realities of the post-pandemic period. We are still dealing with loans taken out to keep the structure functional during the pandemic. Additionally, our leading investor departed during this time, leaving our business no longer supported by external investment. Now, the company needs to be one hundred percent profitable.

Today, all operational aspects of the business are under my management. We have a super lean and fantastic team of six senior employees who handle operational management alongside me. Additionally, we have a wonderful community—the Kaiut community—in Brazil and abroad.

Today, I realize that we need to propagate the Kaiut method. To achieve this, we must embody the method as a community, going beyond just a school and a teacher. My father has successfully impacted this community every day, but we know there are many more people out there who also need this method.

I feel a responsibility to help expand the method's reach. My father excels in the classroom and is arguably the best at what he does. However, he can only transmit his knowledge effectively if the administrative and operational parts are functioning smoothly.

Before, I didn't feel like an heir to anything. My primary goal was simply to make money. However, everything changed when I became a teacher. I discovered the satisfaction of doing work that genuinely helps people. Small, everyday things that are very cool happen and are so rewarding. For instance, one of our teachers had a student, a young woman who struggled to get pregnant. Her pelvic floor was tight, restricting blood flow despite all possible medical treatments. After six months of practicing Kaiut Yoga… pregnant!

Today, I feel like part of a legacy spanning three generations dedicated to health: my grandfather Antonio, my father Francisco, and myself.

The Kaiut Clan—that's how I see its three members, working in harmony, just as they were at the Gramado Summit you witnessed at the beginning of this book. Their synchronized efforts are evident in the collaborative performance of Antonio and Ravi at the Batel school, and Francisco and Ravi, with the latter managing the brand's expansion from their headquarters in Curitiba. Meanwhile, Francisco is engaged in what truly captivates him from his new base in São Paulo, which involves researching, studying, expanding their work, and teaching, both in-person in Brazil and digitally to a global audience.

The transition to the digital world and its integration into Francisco's and the brand's activities was a direct result of the COVID-19 pandemic. Ravi began working strategically on social media, creating, or updating dedicated websites and blogs in both Portuguese and English. This initiative represented a close partnership between father and son, each contributing their unique expertise. It marked a significant turning point.

The matters of schools, expansion, online projects, and courses, these are all very clear to me... but that's all Ravi's work. He wanted to pursue these initiatives, so I do everything possible to support his efforts. I approved many of these endeavors. My focus, on the other hand, is on research, study, and teaching.

During the pandemic, Ravi introduced me to the possibilities of technology, giving me complete freedom to navigate the digital environment. I already had hundreds of lesson plans prepared, with the technical coherence of the method perfectly established. The logic of the method is captured in the basic package of 100 very efficient classes.

I spread all the materials out on my desk and tried to figure it all out. My doubts and challenges surfaced. I thought, "okay, it´s okay... I'll be giving virtual classes to God knows how many people.... only God knows where they will be.... what kind of language will I need to use? How will I present the method effectively?"

I saw it as a terrific opportunity—this is how my mind works, as you already know. I analyzed what other teachers were doing, watched many video classes, and ultimately decided on the pre-recorded format. When the camera operator arrived and asked how many classes I wanted to record, I answered, one hundred!

Actually, I recorded 400 classes: 100 in Portuguese, 100 in English, and an additional 200 that were more complex versions of these basic classes. I also recorded numerous lectures and technical content, and on top of that, I gave live online lectures and workshops.

I set up my first digital course for teacher training, fragmenting the essence of the 100 classes and their theoretical support into a 30-day program. The first thing I did was choose a suitable didactic format. Then, I practiced each digital class and recorded it twice on the same day, first in Portuguese, then in English. This process would evolve over the next seven months.

When I reviewed the first 30 video classes, I realized that the course had excellent content, even by my demanding, perfectionist standards. It wasn't shallow or overly commercial. On the contrary, it had turned out very well.

Then I realized that all the teachers who had been straying— those who held in-person events or classes but missed some sessions due to life changes—coalesced around the online course. This shift allowed me to deliver far more technical content than traditional in-person training ever allowed.

In these cases, what happens?

In an in-person setting, you sit on the floor, which can be uncomfortable and distracting during a technical lecture that lasts an hour. However, online, you need a didactic format that is less physically challenging. You need a chair, a table, a screen, and the ability to focus.

When I realized that online I had more focus and could deliver more information, it was a revelation. While in-person practice events are ideal, I decided then that I would never eliminate the digital format option for our teacher training course.

Any reservations I had about the effectiveness of online practice were dispelled when I observed one of our students. She had taken regular digital classes—not the teacher training course—during the pandemic and later attended in-person classes. Her progress was spectacular, and the results were clearly evident.

Another issue was also resolved. In in-person courses, not all teachers engage in a therapeutic process, and they do not build this place of self-care. They often look to someone else first in order to act.

During the pandemic, I wasn't there in person, and everyone was in lockdown. This forced them to rely on themselves and take initiative. Consequently, the problem solved itself, and I noticed we began to deliver better-prepared teachers to the market.

I realized that I had the opportunity to deliver far more significant content than I had initially imagined. The transition to online teaching was a shocking revelation for me.

A turning point!

The pandemic had more surprises to pull out of its dark, mysterious hat. You know that archetypal figure from myths and comics—the cruel, tragic, and unsettling character, like the Joker in Batman? The one who forces us to confront truths we'd rather avoid? In the midst of horror, this character compels us to look where we don't want to, often pushing us into the shadowy caves of our fears and imagined monsters lurking within the unconscious. We may instinctively turn away, avoiding the discomfort of what lies ahead. But if we dare to face it, if we truly look, beyond the darkness, we might see... a garden?

The pandemic was, for me, like earning a doctorate in my own work. It offered a profound understanding of everything at the next level. The pre-existing knowledge from my classes, my accumulated experience, and everything I had done in yoga all advanced significantly. Understanding the essence of the brand, the work, and the development of the method from the Batel school was crucial.

My understanding of my own method and the technical aspects of things I had intuitively created twenty-something years ago reached a high level of maturation. This is where my current ability to precisely explain what I do, why I do it, and how it works comes from.

I believe that even my understanding of pain evolved. As I entered the pandemic with an injury...

Before the pandemic, my last event in Brazil was a teachers' gathering in Gramado. The night before the opening, I was having fun with my close friend Leandro in the backyard. We were being quite playful, running around having a fruit war. Then it started to rain. As we ran, I stepped on a loose rock. The stone shifted, and I heard a crack. My achillies tendon in my right leg had ruptured completely, creating about a four-centimeter [1.6 inch] separation, as I would later discover.

I went to teach in a wheelchair. It was super interesting because the students had never imagined such a situation. I always had an internal principle: never use a problem as an excuse for why something can't work. Instead, you use the situation, whatever it may be, to make it work.

So, I conducted the class sitting down, either in the wheelchair or perched atop a countertop, as standing was not an option. This limitation pushed me to make the event the best, in terms of verbal instruction, that I had ever done. The fact that I couldn't rely on my body actually made the event better for both the students and me.

There were doctors there who wanted to medicate me and even suggested taking me to a hospital. I told them,

"Guys, I'm not going to medicate myself because if I do, I won't understand what's going on with my body. I can go to a hospital, but only after this event is over."

I researched everything about the injury and returned home without taking anti-inflammatories, painkillers, or anything. When

I arrived, Alissa convinced me to see a doctor. It wasn't about resistance; I saw it as an opportunity to learn something new and take my experience to a new level.

The doctor examined me and said,

"You'll have to undergo surgery. Look, it's separated by four centimeters! Let's prepare. I'm going to immobilize it."

I left the doctor's office with my surgery already scheduled for a few days later. We were already in a pre-pandemic situation, and I didn't have any more events to hold. There was nothing else to do, so I went back home. I took off my orthopedic boot and did yoga.

When the day of the surgery arrived, the doctor took off my boot and said he needed to do one last scan before the operation. I had the scan and when he returned he said,

"I'm not going to operate."

Alissa's jaw dropped,

"What do you mean, doctor?"

"The tendon is healing. I prefer not to operate because it is regenerating. Let's put a cast on it instead."

He also said I couldn't put my weight on my foot at all, even with the cast.

Then, the pandemic truly set in, and we committed to the digital course. So, I had yoga to practice and 400 classes to record.

I asked them to remove the cast and began testing each of my classes.

Remarkably, the classes were what reconstituted the tendon, one hundred percent! There was no recurrence of any issues and no limitation.

As a result of going through that experience, my understanding of the method improved quite substantially.

To this day, people don't believe that it was possible for me to fully recover from a ruptured achillies tendon without surgery or painkillers. All I can say is that: I practice yoga, dealing with pain is part of it. In this case, I focused on reducing inflammation and promoting recovery. And as a result, I ended up better than before!

For others who get themselves in a similar situation, the issue isn't that they lack my experience or knowledge and therefore need to follow the traditional path of medicine. That's not the problem. The problem is that a self-healing process takes effort and dedication. The perspective is different. Many people aren't willing to commit that much. Hospitals are full not because the world is universally sick, but because it's convenient for patients to outsource their health needs. It's a different approach, you know!?

I didn't even see it as a problem. I saw it as an opportunity.

Once again, Francisco takes the less common perspective towards what arises in life. More of the same is coming. I enquire further, the pandemic has brought him many challenges, but also...

Many blessings. Alissa and I were already living together with the children, her children. Then, the pandemic forced us to truly live together as a couple. It turned out to be a perfect thing.

When I was amid frequent travel, living in Curitiba became problematic. I always had to make a connection at the major airport hub in São Paulo. This added two extra days to my trips—one more day outbound and one more day inbound—and resulted in more exhaustion. It was crazy! Even for frequent trips from Curitiba to Porto Alegre, I had to travel via a connection in São Paulo.

You only have to look at the map to understand the absurdity that Francisco is talking about. There may be some convoluted logic in airline flight planning, but for the passenger and the simple geography of the routes, it makes no sense.

Everything passed through São Paulo. So, it made no sense not to be here anymore. Moreover, I have always enjoyed the city, which I felt welcomed me very warmly. So, I started staying here longer from 2015 onward.

Thus, it was only during the pandemic, and with the decision to combine his life with Alissa and her children, that another role for São Paulo emerged on Francisco's horizon: to become his operational base for research and teaching, while Curitiba would remain the operational base for the business with Ravi.

I realized that despite having trained many teachers here in São Paulo, no one had truly embraced the method. No one came forward to start a school. At some point, I understood this is a vital market and wanted to be here. But I wanted it to be myself. I didn't want to be represented by someone else.

In August 2022, still amid the pandemic, but in a less aggressive phase, Ateliê Kaiut Yoga opened in the Pinheiros neighborhood. This marked the first venture in partnership with Alissa, now his partner in both life and this significant business undertaking.

Here, Francisco conducts in-person classes exclusively, every workday, week after week, and often five times a day, with few breaks throughout the year. This is also where he records most of his digital classes and events, and where he holds real-time online meetings with teachers in training both in Brazil and abroad.

During the research period for this book, real characters from this story who came to Brazil for further development as teachers passed through this room—Kristin Savory, Darvin Ayre, and Yvonne Mosser, twice, on the second visit accompanied by her son and business partner, Cliff.

If you recall we were here, in Ateliê in chapter nine, as people settled into class with their legs up the wall. You've traveled through so many places in this narrative, starting with the Summit in Gramado, that it's understandable if you've forgotten you've been here before.

If you came by car this time, hand it over to Ademir, the valet. Parking is complimentary. Ademir's an attentive, helpful, and nice guy. His teenage daughter, Larissa, recently started working at the school as a receptionist too. If not Larissa, Adriana the other friendly receptionist and teacher of the method may greet you.

Welcome. The door is open.

19

Master

Imagine in front of you a large virtual projection screen. This advanced technology transports and immerses you into a new reality, into the classroom, offering a glimpse into Francisco's world, his method, and the vibrant Kaiut Yoga community.

Whether you're a teacher, practitioner, or visitor—here out of curiosity, skepticism, or what feels like coincidence—you are invited to take a moment. Lie down on the mat with your head resting on the bolster, legs up against the wall.

This is the perfect opportunity to pause and experience something that could be transformative, whether in small or significant ways. Notice how the story unfolds for you—the emotions it stirs, the thoughts it provokes, and the impact it might quietly have on your body.

As we near the end of this narrative journey, we first need to hear from a few more voices within the Kaiut community, individuals who have traveled a similar path and whose testimonials offer further glimpses into the profound impact of this method. Their reflections connect the threads of this story, bridging the historical and thematic arcs of this journey, adding new dimensions to its meaning.

Although of course, we will return to Francisco, to hear his final words at the Gramado Summit—the place where our journey began. His reflections will draw this book to a close, but may also perhaps leave room for more... But first, more from the community.

Diana Witczak trained as a teacher when she was 38 years old, during the pregnancy of her second child, Inácio. She traveled 345 miles (565 kms) by bus to Gramado, spending entire nights on the road to and from every weekend training session. She lives in Doutor Maurício Cardoso, a small town with a population of only 4,470 inhabitants (in 2022), located on the banks of the Uruguay River in the northwest of Rio Grande do Sul, near the border with Argentina. Her licensed school serves as an example of the geographical extremes to which the method has reached within the country and highlights the unique circumstances of its expansion into Deep Brazil.

The city has been quite resistant to yoga, but I'm working on opening people's minds to challenge the paradigms and beliefs that lead to prejudice. I'm striving to demonstrate that with Kaiut Yoga it is possible to age without the deterioration commonly associated with getting older.

In the beginning, only women were practicing. Now, I have nine men attending classes, including my father. I ran a promotion offering a free month for husbands, and several of them continued after the trial. One of them, who had undergone spinal surgery, resisted his doctor's advice to stop doing yoga. He hasn't missed a single class since and says he feels better every day.

I have 70 private students, plus four groups of 15 people each, whose classes are funded by the municipality. Now, the City Hall is discussing a new agreement with me, as they want to sponsor classes for communities in the interior of the municipality that have been requesting yoga.

From the Gramado Summit, two further voices recount how they overcame significant health challenges through their practice.

Neiva Votto experienced a psychiatric breakdown triggered, as she believes, by accumulated stress primarily due to her husband's sigmoid colon cancer. He spent two months in agony, barely sleeping, and she was constantly helping in the emergency room with his hemorrhagic condition, seeking a doctor in Argentina, and following through with the surgeries. This situation led to a loss of her ability to work, heavily impacting family relationships, and requiring psychiatric support and medication.

Everything changed when she climbed the mountain for the first time—as she describes it, to attend Francisco's training course in Gramado. The first class felt like a balm, transforming her entirely. It was her turning point.

The first lesson felt like a response to a scream that had been stuck in my throat. I felt heard. Everything Francisco said seemed to be directed at me. His determined speech led me to a place of self-awareness and introspection. It was exactly what I needed.

Cecília Salek, a Kaiut Yoga teacher in Rio de Janeiro, balances the demands of her busy urban life as a mother of three and a production engineer with 15 years of experience in the telecommunications industry by turning to daily yoga practice. She shares that this practice helps her manage the stress she has carried since the age of 13, when she was diagnosed with a bone cyst at the head of her left femur. That stress, compounded by years of physical strain and a rupture of the anterior cruciate ligament in her left knee—accompanied by looming warnings of mandatory surgery—began to ease at age 45, when she discovered Kaiut Yoga after trying conventional yoga for some time.

At the Gramado Summit, Cecília recounted an extraordinary moment. A recent MRI, taken just months before the event, prompted her to question the results. Her orthopedist, however, assured her, "The exam is correct. You no longer have a bone injury in your left hip. It has completely reconstituted. It's almost a miracle. You've been blessed."

From the Summit, the story shifts to São Paulo, where another pair of students, Marise and Celso Cipriani, share their journey with the method—a journey spanning continents and profound life changes.

When living in Boulder, Marise first heard about Francisco's visit from their friends David and Helena Bolduc. Despite her background in conventional yoga and a keen interest in alternative health paths, she initially hesitated to attend. They had said, "It's a different type of yoga," which didn't spark her interest at the time.

Eventually, Marise attended a session and encouraged her husband Celso to join her.

"It's good for you, Celso. It works like mental hygiene."

His response was firm,

"I don't need it. I have my own mental hygiene—hunting and fishing. I'm getting back to it after all those years dealing with Transbrasil."

Marise's father, Omar Fontana, was the iconic founder of Transbrasil, once the third-largest airline in Brazil. Celso served as the company's CEO during its turbulent final years, culminating in its involuntary bankruptcy in 2002. The process, which involved a legal battle with General Electric over aircraft leasing, placed immense stress on Celso, taking a significant toll on his health.

The couple once considered partnering with Francisco to open a Kaiut Yoga school in Boulder. However, Marise's commitments to a large real estate and leisure business in Colorado demanded her full attention, and the partnership didn't materialize.

Their connection with Francisco deepened after his return to Brazil, particularly when he lived in Campinas, São Paulo, and later when he opened the São Paulo studio. Marise became a regular student, and Celso joined classes whenever his frequent business trips allowed. Now based in São Paulo, Celso travels extensively, often to the northern state of Amapá, but remains a dedicated practitioner when his schedule permits.

In the classroom, Celso is known for his positive energy and his stories of overcoming challenges through Francisco's method. He recalls one particularly memorable incident when he arrived in a wheelchair. After two hours of consultation and practice, he was able to stand up and leave feeling noticeably better.

When I arrive at class, I often joke, "for God's sake, am I paying to come here and suffer!?" But by the time the practice is over, my body and mind are ecstatic. I leave feeling like I'm walking on clouds. That's when I realize that the work is truly working!

You can see that the method is indeed working well for students attending the new classes in São Paulo. Take Giullia Della Monica, for instance, a 24-year-old business administrator and environmental activist. She joined the classes with a rare herniated vertebral disc for someone her age, a rupture of eighty percent of a disc in her spine.

I had my first injury, followed by a second one. Medical treatment was not resolving the issue. During my first consultation, Francisco described my condition impressively. He discussed problems related to my central nervous system and my issues with cramps and menstruation. He also mentioned my hypersensitivity just by looking at my eyes, noting that my pupils are always dilated because I am constantly in a state of emergency, reacting to stress differently than others. He said this has consequences because I internalize a lot of my body's stress. He explained that numerous traumas from my life have been accumulating in my body since childhood, and the catalyst for the crisis was the rupture of the disc.

The crisis was at its peak when I arrived for my first classes. I couldn't stand for more than five minutes, walk, or drive. Someone had to help me out of the car and into the room. During the first month, I took the classes on a stretcher.

Now, two months later, I can stand and walk again. Though I still experience some pain, I can engage in activities more freely. Francisco tells me that this is the point where my treatment truly begins. Before, I was just managing the crisis. Now, the treatment can proceed in a systemic and structured way.

You now catch a glimpse of Francisco entering the room out of the corner of your eye. Or perhaps he was there from the beginning, unnoticed. You suspect he's about to speak soon. But for now, your attention remains captivated by the voices of the community.

Melanie Marquetti is the newest member of the Batel school teaching team, in Curitiba. She turned to yoga due to a longstanding issue with spondylolisthesis, a condition involving spinal misalignment, nerve compression, and, in her case, a fracture in the lumbar vertebrae L4 and L5. Melanie arrived with a love-hate relationship with Kaiut Yoga.

> Every time I picked up that exercise block in class, I wanted to throw it at the wall. I knew it would lead me to a level of pain far beyond my tolerance. It was always pain and crying. I would leave the class in tears.

Melanie just ran away on the first day, but she came back the next. The desire to find a light at the end of the tunnel of her intense suffering made her believe that this could be the place.

However, her journey was anything but linear. Melanie moved to different cities, endured a car accident, underwent surgery, and faced a marital breakdown. Yet, she persisted. She eventually resumed her practice and completed her teacher training in Curitiba while living in Blumenau, Santa Catarina, 150 miles (243 kms) away. During this time, she felt driven by what she considers the Holy Spirit to help others and took up volunteering in a community kitchen for those in need. This led her to wonder what more she could do.

The answer came through a surprising invitation from a private student, a partner at an integrative medicine clinic, who asked her to teach Kaiut Yoga classes there. So, in the middle of the pandemic in October 2020, Melanie introduced the method to the city. In another twist of fate, she returned to Curitiba in January 2023 and received an informal internship offer from Francisco, followed by an invitation to join the teaching staff at the Batel school, where she began teaching in April.

And after this all this, how does she now see Francisco?

He's a genius. As a teacher, he can be tough, and sometimes we, as students, just want to feel welcomed. However, it's through this tough stance that he enables us to transform. He has an incredible ability to extract the best from each of us.

Well, he's here now. You can feel his presence. However, the final mini testimony is about to unfold and draw your attention. It touches on a quality that many may associate with Francisco but hesitate to articulate—perhaps out of a desire to avoid any connotation of idolatry or a misinterpretation of the often-misunderstood concept of a *guru*. One person, however, articulates this quality with perfect clarity: Frances Rose Feder.

A practitioner in São Paulo, Frances has long been involved with the world of Sacred Circle Dances, a deep exploration of body and movement. She also happens to be the informal godmother of this book—for reasons you're about to discover. Her insight emerged during a week of classes with Francisco at Lapinha Spa, one of Brazil's top integrative health and medical retreats, located 49 miles (80 kms) south of Curitiba airport.

At the closing session of the event, Frances shared her thoughts with Francisco and the group:

For me, this event was surprising and impactful, a key moment of change in my life. I arrived with limitations that had plagued me for the last seven years. Initially, I fell and tore my meniscus, leading to arthritis and various hip complications. I began to limp and gained more weight—an issue I already struggled with—which affected my lumbar region. This compensation grew into a profound limitation, bringing with it a deep sadness. A sadness over lost time, especially since I'm at an age where I can't afford to waste time.

But then an extraordinarily strong insight came to me, a deep, intuitive trust in what you've done and said here, Francisco. The realization that we often protect the pain, and not ourselves, struck me profoundly. So, I committed to the work. I didn't just do what I usually do, which is overthink things.

I have worked with many leading figures in the area of self-knowledge and translated for many of them. There are a lot of good people and excellent teachers, but very few true masters. For me, it is exceedingly difficult to consider someone a master. I have knowledge, content, and a critical mind. But you, Francisco, stood out from the first day. You are a master.

There are many feelings for the excellence of your work. But the main one and what sums it all up is gratitude. Deep gratitude.

So, how is Frances the spontaneous godmother of this project?

Frances—someone very dear to my heart—returned to São Paulo inspired. She spoke glowingly of Francisco and the method, vowing to enroll at the new studio as soon as it opened. She also encouraged me to join, and I agreed.

Knowing my skill as a writer with a knack for telling stories of transformative lives, she suggested that the story of Francisco and his method deserved a narrative of the highest quality. She reached out to Alissa, who had already considered the idea of a biography. Together, they arranged a lunch for the three of us to present the idea to Francisco. As you might have guessed, convincing him was a success and the result is the very story you're now holding in your hands.

So, now I place myself in the room with you and everyone else. You can lower your legs, rest your spine, relax your nervous system, and calm your breathing. We all sit, each on our own mat, in whatever way feels comfortable, cross-legged, or not.

There you see him. And the others—Ravi, Bruna, Antonio, and Alissa. Standing at the front of the room, Francisco. No, he doesn't have the mate gourd in his hands. He is holding Bento, preparing to deliver his closing remarks on keys to sustainable practice and a vision for the future.

Movement is life. Transmutation is consciousness. Mastery is allowing Nature to bring out the best of your potential as a divine human being. Pain in the body, mind, and heart serves as the portal to transcendence, to immanence, to everything.

And what about the nature and role of perception in all this? To perceive is to be present in the whole. This means being aware of your body... movement... sensations... emotions... and all the stimuli around you... processing everything in an integral, systemic, and holistic way. You are guided to be sensitive to everything, without judgment.

When you observe and connect with long-standing pain without making value judgments, you initiate a therapeutic process. This triggers a state of calm, activating the parasympathetic nervous system, that leads to growth, repair, and an anti-inflammatory response. The more you engage in this process grounded in nonjudgmental perception, your understanding deepens, and the body no longer needs to react unproductively.

The transmutation of pain arises from the awareness a person gains about their own situation. Pain carries within it the seed of the solution. While not all pain will respond without medical or surgical intervention, I have never encountered pain that does not respond to acceptance. Pain needs to be seen, accepted, welcomed, and transmuted. The region of the body that suffers pain feels as if it has been excluded from the natural wholeness of which it is a part. Consequently, it suffers more. It is essential to bring this region back into contact with the ancestral wisdom of self-perception. The state of presence generated by the method has a physical anchor, which is the body.

As I've stated, I define yoga as a chronic state of presence with emotional coherence, mirroring the way Nature operates. In practice, in the classroom, the construction of this state of presence requires the teacher to guide students in feeling, rather than analyzing, interpreting, judging, or controlling. This approach puts the active, thinking, and analytical mind on stand-by.

A collective intelligence takes over and determines that movement will occur. Upon observation, you see that movement does not originate from a single being, it simultaneously emerges from several individuals who are neither seeing nor in contact with each other.

So, teaching Kaiut Yoga integrates all human essences and existences into a collective flow state. This shared flow state enables us to move away from our limitations more quickly and is highly healing.

Furthermore, this idea that there is a separation between body and mind is wrong. There is no separation between body and mind. In the brain, we have a map of the body located in the prefrontal cortex. This map shrinks when the body is used less and expands when its use is consistent and safe.

Science already knows that more yoga equals less Alzheimer's. Why is this? The correct use of the body impacts the brain's image of the body. When this image is well nourished by regular use of the *body—remaining clear, sharp, and transparent—it helps ensure that the brain stays healthier. And vice versa.*

To use the body and brain properly, you must have the right intention. For example, many people in the world of dance who experience pain come to yoga, claiming to be highly aware of their bodies. But there is no body awareness there!

As I've also touched on already, the brain works like Aladdin's Lamp, granting unlimited wishes. Neuroplastically, it constantly finds compensatory routes to overcome problems and provide you with what you want in the moment. As a dancer, my desire is to perform impeccably for the audience and critics. I seek to know my body position in space, movement, aesthetics, form, lightness, and harmony. However, I do not prioritize health, embodied presence, neural reconnection, or an expanded brain map because performance takes precedence over functionality. The outcome then in terms of true health is different.

Intention is fundamental. Thus, awareness of intention is key.

Understanding the importance of full movement of the hip joint is equally essential. It is the energetic crank turning the wheel of life. The hip connects the pelvis, spine, and lower limbs, and is a major transit hub and access point to the lymphatic system, circulatory system, and major nerve pathways. Healthy, organized movement in the hip joint is critical for the entire body to operate smoothly.

Walking, for instance, provides a gentle massage to the joints and muscles of the entire body, affecting everything from the pelvis downwards and upwards to the shoulders and head. The hip is also intimately related to the entire pelvic region. Thus, issues with the hip have a direct impact on the muscles and health of the pelvic floor. When this is compromised issues concerning sexuality, fertility, bladder function, and prostate health can arise.

Conveniently, in classical medicine, an individual with hip pain is often told that they have a straightforward orthopedic problem. They may not realize that an invasive procedure could systemically compromise the entire health of the region and beyond. People are conditioned to believe in a separation between one aspect and another; that problems are isolated.

However, everything is linked, connected. Male pelvic floor problems, while less obvious, are just as common as female pelvic floor issues and are linked to prostate problems, sexual potency, and numerous other discomforts. Due to distorted ideas in our society however, we no longer see the hip for its primary function—as the engine of life.

At the beginning of developing the method, I analyzed and worked with many students who were athletes, soccer players, and martial art fighters. When they came in complaining of back and knee pain, I noticed that the apparent strength of many of their muscles concealed underlying weaknesses. These muscles lacked stability and joint mobility.

I looked at those big guys with strong shoulders and wondered, 'what's weak? What is in disharmony? What is out of proportion?' The answer was always the same: the feet!

This realization has produced remarkable results. I noticed that many women with urinary incontinence problems, due to a compromised pelvic floor, experienced rapid improvements after a sequence of foot exercises. Then I understood... "whoa! An unlocked foot initiates systemic unblocking and natural toning of the entire structure of the legs and pelvis." This made me realize that the body's mechanism and overall health cannot be understood through isolated segments.

But then, what is the origin of the hidden fragility in one of these super strong guys?

It is the culture of specialization and segmented understanding. Specialization leads to the underutilization of certain angles in each joint. Overused angles might get injured, but you don't suffer from what you do, you suffer from what you don't do. It is the underused angles, those you don't notice or use, which will lead to issues and injury, as is it those areas and angles that age very quickly.

That's what's happening to everyone because everybody is aging at the hip. The human pelvis has been suffering the consequences of the Industrial Revolution for generations. Our species is no longer as active as it once was. Our species is no longer moving. Generations upon generations spend their lives sitting.

It's not that the species inherently handles stress poorly. It's that we cope badly with stress when our bodies don't move in the right way. Consequently, the human pelvis, which is deteriorating, is a major area of suffering. Of all our structures, the pelvis is perhaps the one most contradicted by modern life. This has led to a pandemic of low back pain, visceral disorders, prostate issues, and problems with the womb, ovaries, and bladder.

So again, we return to the question of rescue? How do we rescue our health; everything we've lost?

And again, I reassert that we need to start at the feet. The feet rarely cause you to suffer today. Instead, they generate systemic discomfort that is often silent. Everything that happens in the feet subtly echoes upwards, creating a resonance between the plantar, pelvic and shoulder girdles. These three girdles seek balance from a gravitational perspective, transferring forces through muscles and fascia.

That's why I focus so much on ground-based work. In doing so, we neutralize the impact of gravity on the standing body. On the ground, we can achieve a greater depth of access and facilitate effective movement.

We continue sitting on mats on the floor, supported by bolsters or not. Absorbed by this stream of knowledge and wisdom from Francisco.

Curiosity gets the better of me, I want to know Francisco's projection of the future, both immediate and longer term.

For me, the future is closely tied to the classroom. Here in São Paulo, as in all the places where I have worked, there is nothing quite like what I do. It's a whole new concept.

As you know, I am not opposed to doctors or the pharmaceutical industry. However, these two forces often dominate discussions about health, even though their fundamental focus is not truly on health itself. At times, their priorities are commercial; at other times, they revolve around the management of disease. I find this quite questionable.

I've come to recognize a critical gap—a space unoccupied by science or complementary therapies. It is the space for rescuing health from a completely natural perspective, a space free from conflict and subservience to any external agenda. This is where my practice and work belong: restoring health naturally, intelligently, and sustainably. I believe this has become truly clear in my return to the classroom, both in-person and online, after the pandemic.

The market and the people strongly need the resource I provide. I believe this is reflected in the success of the Ateliê Kaiut Yoga here in

São Paulo. We are already completely booked, with a waiting list for almost every class. When we move to the new headquarters, which will be a school accommodating 42 students, I think we will quickly face the same issue of lack of space.

Part of this demand stems from my experience, but another significant factor is the public's unmet need for a simple, natural, and intelligent resource that delivers sustainable, authentic health benefits.

I want to expand this work by continuing to deliver physical and structural improvements, pain relief, functional recovery, and enhanced metabolic and mental health. My goal is to produce an abundance of meaningful results. Over the next 30 years, I want to dedicate myself fully to the classroom, helping people age under the influence of my method. By doing so, I hope to create a lasting body of work that demonstrates, in real and measurable ways, how aging can be profoundly improved for the general population. I aim to hand over 30 years of method development to the same group of people, so that the recorded information about aging in this way becomes very palpable and beneficial for the general population.

I know that Ravi has a desire to focus more on the educational aspect within our commercial world. That's fine, but as for me, I now give myself the right to be a mad scientist in a laboratory, doing only what I love, with the people I enjoy working with, and nourishing schools and teachers with this information.

Other initiatives?

Upon completion of the original version of this book you are reading now, there will be significant online events in the United States and Brazil. Already fully booked, these are expected to be the most major events in Francisco's career to date. Additionally, there will be a Summit in Curitiba and a major intensive practice event in Rio Grande do Sul. The opening of the first licensed school in Portugal in the works, and negotiations are underway for the first school in Italy.

In the area of disseminating knowledge about the method, following the numerous ebooks on specific topics such as Alzheimer's, epigenetics, gut health, and yoga for men, Francisco has decided to record 30 hours of lectures in Portuguese and 30 hours in English. These will be compiled into a comprehensive technical book.

Francisco is incredibly pleased with the growth of schools in an increasingly well-structured manner. He acknowledges that Ravi is doing an excellent job in this regard. He also appreciates that the teachers involved in this expansion are now more connected, involved, and dedicated to their own process of continuous education.

Why is this good?

Because it gives me a lot of freedom. With fewer events and less travel, there are fewer distractions, allowing me to spend more time in the classroom. This enables me to fully commit to my life's purpose.

After this, Francisco is silent for a minute. We all remain silent.

He returns Bento to his mother's arms. Bento's destiny is yet to play out. I wish good health and wisdom for this tender child, perhaps such a future is ensured given he is nourished from an early age by the healthy and constructive energy field of the larger environment where he was blessed to be born—the Kaiut clan and Kaiut Yoga. Who knows, he might grow to the full potential of a mutable human being, reaching levels of excellence in the species that we cannot even imagine today.

Francisco then speaks in a serene voice—his words aligned with my own, as this narrative nears its end.

Thank you everyone. As you conclude your practice, carry this state of calm—a relaxed nervous system, a clear mind, and a sense of peace—into the rest of your day or use it to set the foundation for a restful, restorative night's sleep.

Then, standing, he performs the mudra, joining the palms of his hands at the center of his chest.

We do the same, sitting wherever we are. In unison, we all greet each other—children of the stars, blessed creatures of the mystery of life—quietly filled with gratitude for bearing witness to this extraordinary creation. A practice with the power to nurture health, vitality, and longevity. Kaiut Yoga.

Namaste.

The Source of The Elixir

"Everything vibrates, nothing is still, everything moves.
Everything is composed of Spirit vibrating at a certain frequency.
The three characteristics of vibration: order, quality, orientation."

Vibration Principle,
attributed to Hermes Trismegistus.

Seventy minutes, that's how long Francisco's regular class lasts. He conducts in-person classes at Ateliê three times a day on Mondays and Wednesdays, five times a day on Tuesdays and Thursdays, and twice on Fridays. On Tuesdays and Thursdays, the first class begins at six-fifty in the morning, and the last one starts at half past seven in the evening.

He is punctual. Classes start on time and end on time. His understanding of conducting each class, the duration of each position, and the relaxation period at the end are impressive. The whole thing runs smoothly, like clockwork.

His work drive is intense. In addition to these 18 weekly classes, he conducts an online live class in Portuguese for the teacher training course every Monday, which often exceeds two hours in duration. On Wednesdays, he teaches in English for the international teachers-in-training.

This is his basic routine scheduled for the entire year of 2024. Interspersed with this program are extra activities such as events like the Summit, newsletter production, strategic planning and management meetings, addressing specific questions from certified teachers, consultations with individual students, and continuous study and research on topics of interest to him.

He makes few professional trips, preferring to concentrate his activities in São Paulo. He reserves rare occasions for activities in Curitiba, other parts of the country, or abroad, usually at licensed Kaiut Yoga schools.

Family trips, however, are another story. For instance, he visits Curitiba to celebrate the birth of Ravi and Bruna's second child, Franco. And will venture further afield to enjoy school holidays with Alissa and the children.

Today is Saturday, a day dedicated to cleaning at Ateliê. Francisco is super busy but remains at home, within walking distance of the school, engaging in an activity that brings him a lot of satisfaction outside of work.

Meanwhile, Alissa is at the children's school, accompanying Pietra to a children's party. Filipo is here at home, ready to leave, wearing a flashy blue Brazilian national soccer team jersey, official uniform, with a ball in his hands and sneakers on his feet. He is going to the same party but plans to play soccer. He prefers sneakers over boots.

Francisco apologizes for the minor inconvenience, explaining with a smile that the house is in domestic chaos due to a last-minute change in the school's schedule. However, he needs to take Filipo there, as the boy is still too young to be allowed on the streets alone.

Francisco returns shortly. Then he sits on the floor, legs crossed, knees dropped to the sides, and feet touching the mat. He's doing... Kaiut Yoga.

On his right knee are the accessories he uses in classes: sandbags weighing about six and half pounds (3 kgs) each. I note that in the classroom Francisco typically works with only one bag per student, but here, he has four on his knee. I joke and tease him,

"It's because you're a teacher and need more strength, right?"

He lets out a quick laugh, accepting the unexpected joke and getting into the spirit of it.

Actually, I usually use six. I tend to work with a lot of weight, but I wanted a slightly lighter practice today, so I'm only using four...

The homely, relaxed atmosphere is conducive to Francisco engaging in sincere reflection on the balance of his life—encompassing the story of the individual, Francisco, and his work, the method.

There is the ongoing construction of his first and only school in São Paulo, which will serve as the administrative and operational headquarters for his activities. He will be the exclusive on-site teacher there. The school will welcome practicing students and teachers from Brazil and abroad for special teacher training programs. Additionally, many events will be streamed online from this location. It's situated on Groenlândia Street, a prime area of the city, close to his current location.

I want to counterpoint what I said at the beginning of our conversation, at the start of the book: that I lived in a rigid, reactive, traumatized inner universe.

This is relevant to revisit because, to a large extent, we are shaped by our past. However, at some point, we need to make the choice to become different, to not just be a product of our history, you know?

I see how much yoga is a tool that creates conditions for transformation in a magical way. Yoga is a healing art. I say this because I see changes not only in my body but also in my mental patterns—my way of thinking, my perspective on life, and my actions. I see how this inner universe has transformed, creating a harmonious manifestation in my surroundings, free from conflicts and tensions, you know? This is what the Principle of Correspondence speaks to: this relationship between inside and the outside; In turn, I have come to review my life from the perspective of self-responsibility.

When reflecting on my divorce from Luciana, I realize that much of what generated that stormy situation stemmed from within me, from my conscious mind or even unconscious universe. It was, in fact, a manifestation of my inner state.

This also relates to my parent's attitude when my first child Samantha was born. Overall, this was another traumatic event in my life. Some things in me were never the same again. While the previous incident left a big wound, Samantha's birth left a cut just as deep, if not deeper.

While dealing with an unplanned teenage pregnancy is complicated enough, it was seeing my parents' act in such a harsh and extremely prejudiced way that was further shocking. Both my father and mother displayed prejudice and a lot of machismo. For me, it was unfortunate and disappointing to witness their attitude and see more of who they were and where they had come from. I understand that they wanted to protect me, but the tools they used were prejudice and judgment.

However, later, as an adult, this experience shaped my way of interacting with life: I made it a point not to judge or operate from a prejudiced belief system. This is a crucial part of my career and in the development of teachers. To observe without judgment, under any circumstances, no matter what appears in front of you. The teacher simply operates from the reality at hand, without judgment, and strives to make the best of it.

So, despite the difficulty and pain, despair, anguish, and a lot of fear, at that time as a teenager, it was incredibly good that it happened the way it did. I have a friend who uses a phrase that I really appreciate: "A child is always a goal worth pursuing. There's never a wrong time for it to happen." A child always adds to our journey, you know?

About Luciana... I was the one who brought this person into my life. As much as it may be convenient during a divorce, conflict, and pain to blame the other person or find in them the reason for our suffering, or to feel ashamed of what happened or blame ourselves, that is not the way. I understood that I placed her there, in my life, for better or for worse.

I also ended up very frustrated, hurt, and anguished, experiencing strong feelings of despair during the episode of Malu's loss. But on the other hand, it strengthened me enormously. It was the first significant moment when I stopped merely existing and began seeking deeper spiritual values.

And, in the case of the first yoga school I attended and worked at, I was stepping into the adult world of work. It was my first foray into the professional realm, interacting with people, doing business, and forming associations. I see that, in a way, they provided me with a gateway to the world of yoga. But in another sense, I also chose a path that involved being deceived. Thankfully, today, the people I associate with have a completely different nature. These experiences taught me a vital lesson about the vibrational essence of existence.

I understood that self-responsibility is a decisive step. Only through self-responsibility do we realize that the life around us directly reflects the life within us—as much as we might want to ascribe responsibility to other circumstances or people. This holds for how we often think and speak about health: we can find explanations, point fingers, assign blame, and judge others for their health problems and pain. But at some point we have to embrace self-responsibility. This self-responsibility—not as a burden but as a testament to the human capacity to change frequency—is very important.
In this matter of health and life, yoga is one place we can take up this journey of self-responsibility.

What excites me most about yoga today is the vibrational empowerment
it provides. Through yoga, you can transform—you can stop vibrating from the subconscious influences of your past, whether shaped by your upbringing, education, or trauma. Yoga allows you to vibrate through and transform all these layers—it allows you to make new and different choices, find balance, and ultimately live from a more empowered place. Choosing to practice yoga for several hours a day ultimately means choosing better health, harmonious relationships, and prosperous work.

So, at the end of the day, life is not what happened to me. It is what I chose to make of it.

About the Authors

Francisco Kaiut

Yoga teacher. Chiropractor. Visionary. Mentor.

Founder of the Kaiut Yoga method, Francisco revolutionizes yoga by reconnecting it with its ancestral roots and infusing it with modern wisdom. His approach liberates yoga from the excessive mysticism found in some practices and the exaggerated commercialism seen in fitness-driven approaches. This inclusive style of yoga is designed for everyone, adaptable to the pace and capacity of each individual.

Based in São Paulo, Francisco works both within Brazil and internationally, with a notable presence in the United States. He is committed to promoting, teaching, and sharing his legacy, which transcends cultural and niche boundaries.

kaiutyoga.com.br

Edvaldo Pereira Lima

Writer. Journalist. Biographer. Teacher.

As the creator of the Advanced Literary Journalism method, Edvaldo Pereira Lima merges the art of storytelling with the authenticity of nonfiction literature. His transdisciplinary approach opens fresh perspectives, enhancing our understanding by tapping into our innate wisdom.

His biographical narratives often spotlight remarkable individuals who have a transformative impact on the world—like Francisco.

edvaldopereiralima.com.br

Title	Journey to the Heart of Pain: life story(ies) and the yoga that transforms (them)
Layout	US Trade 6 in x 9 in
Text typography	Minion Pro
Title Typography	Libre Baskerville
Layout	Israel Dias de Oliveira

www.ingramcontent.com/pod-product-compliance
Lightning Source LLC
Chambersburg PA
CBHW050332270326
41926CB00016B/3421

9 786501 327228